Selected Topics in Facial Nerve Disorders

Edited by Isam Al-Zwaini and Mohammed Jalal Hussein

Published in London, United Kingdom

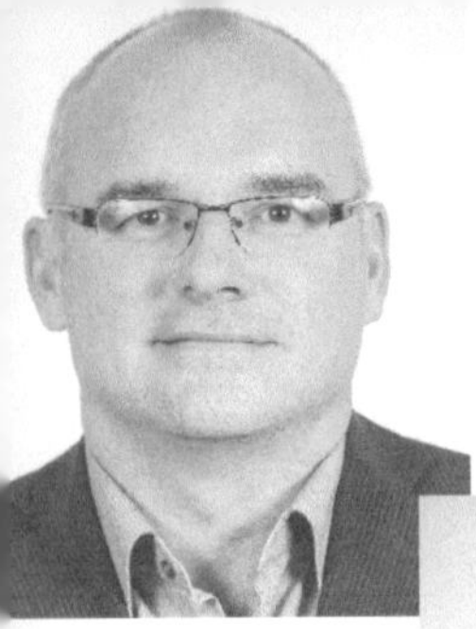
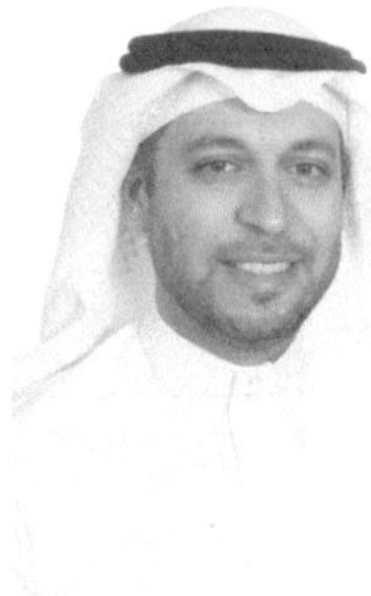
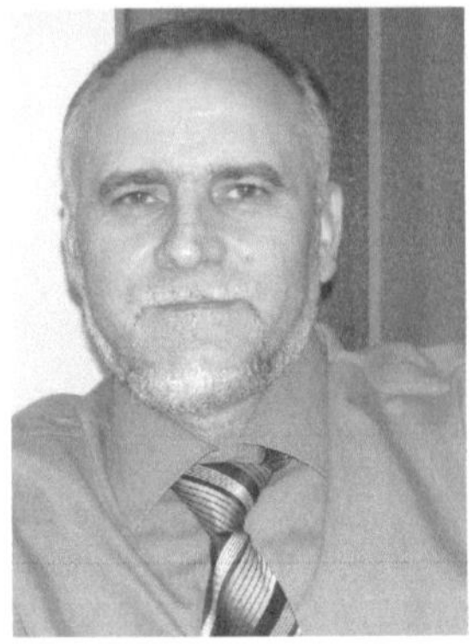
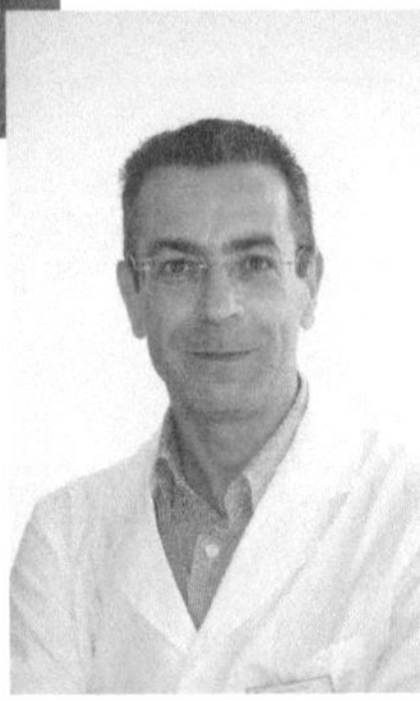
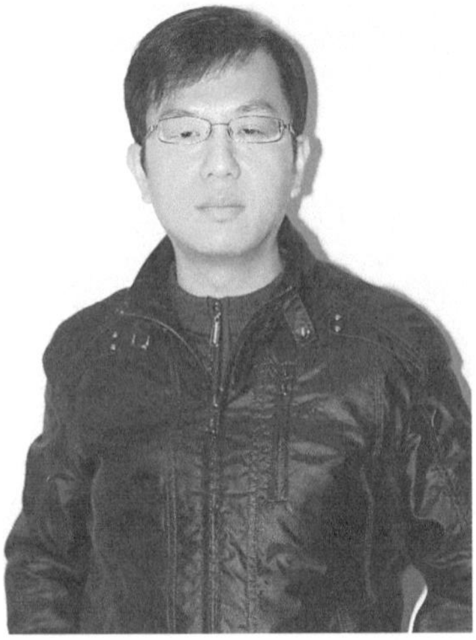
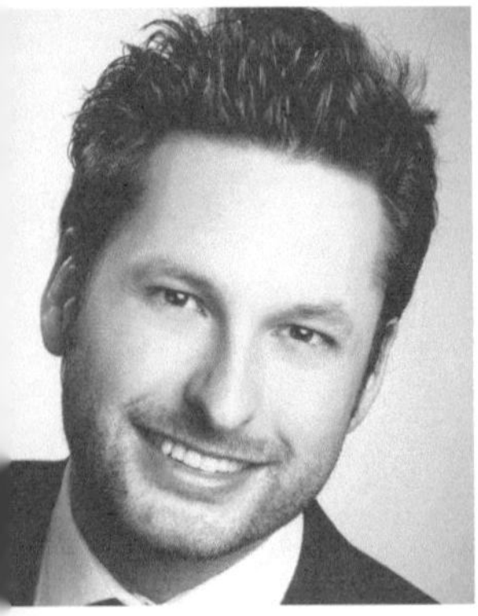
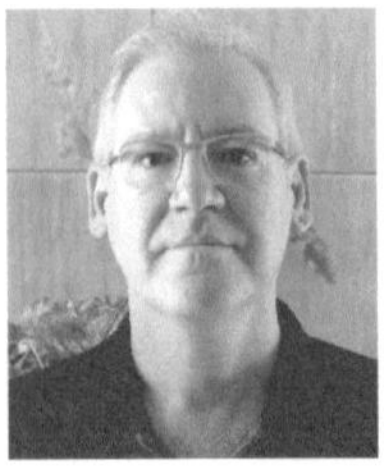

IntechOpen

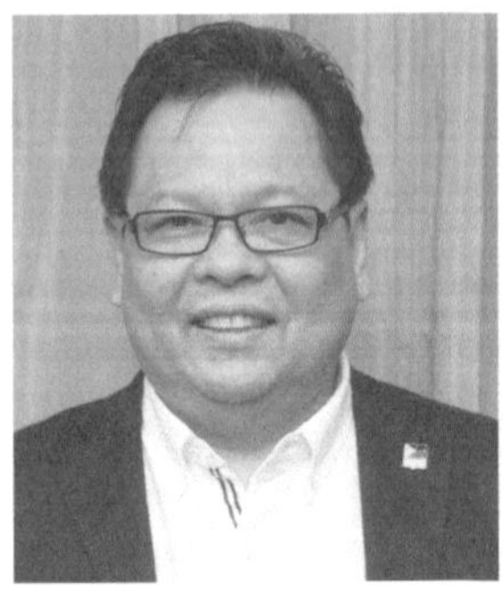
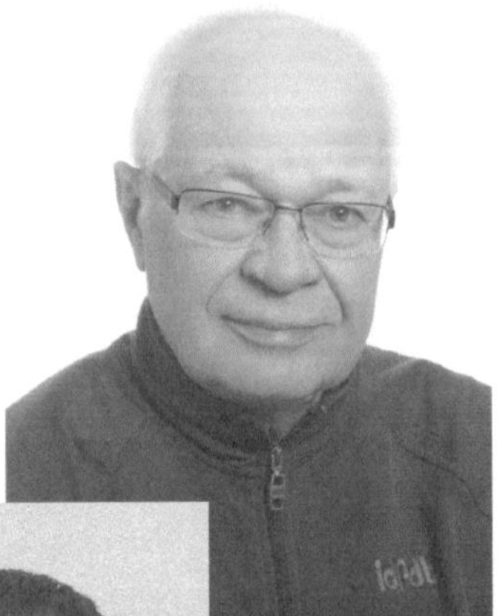
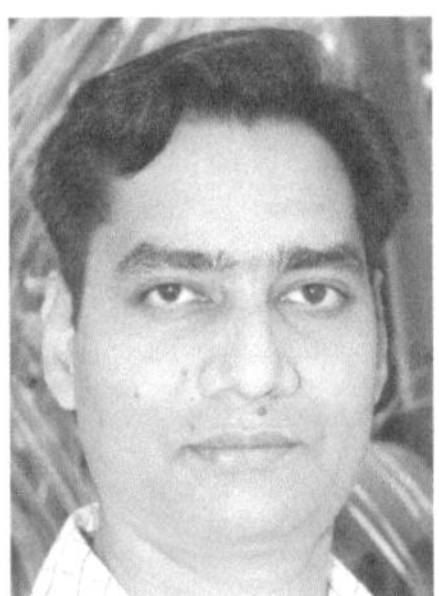
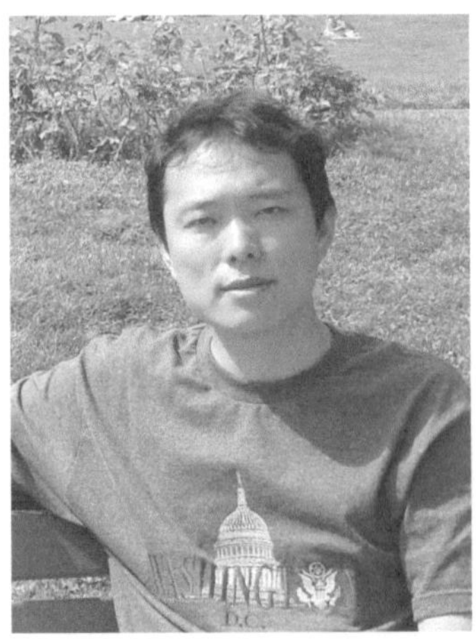
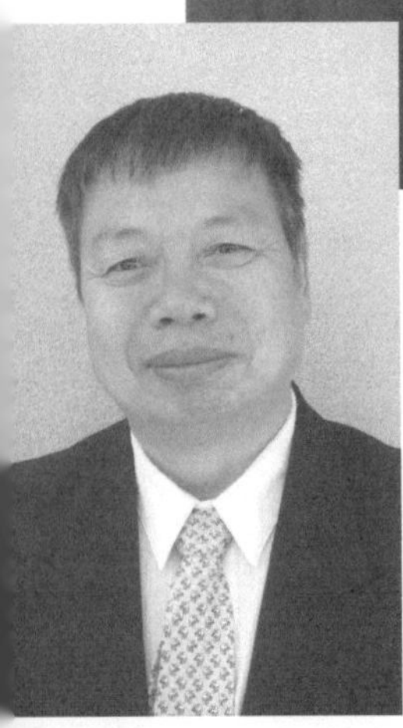
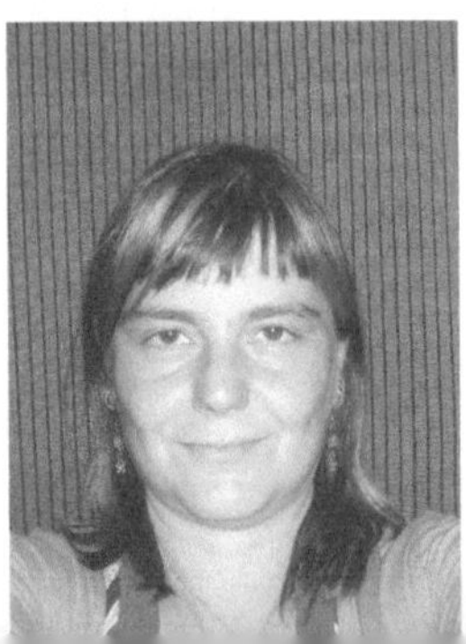

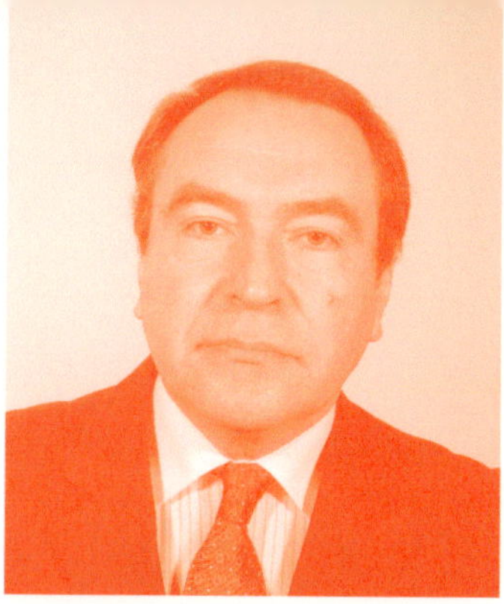
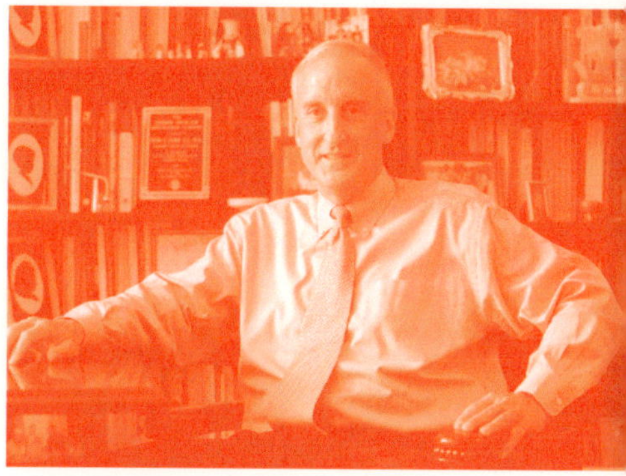
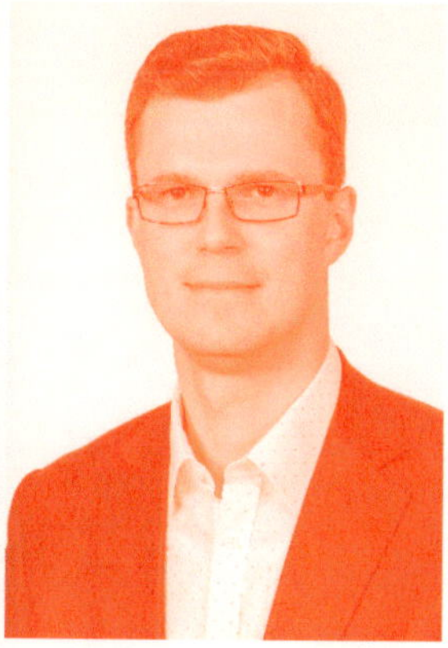
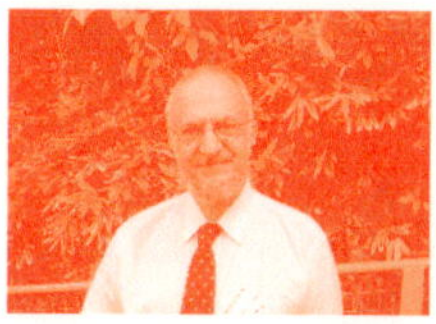
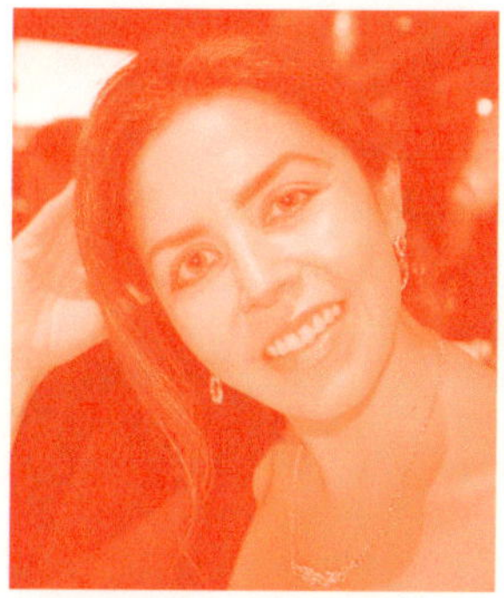

Supporting open minds since 2005

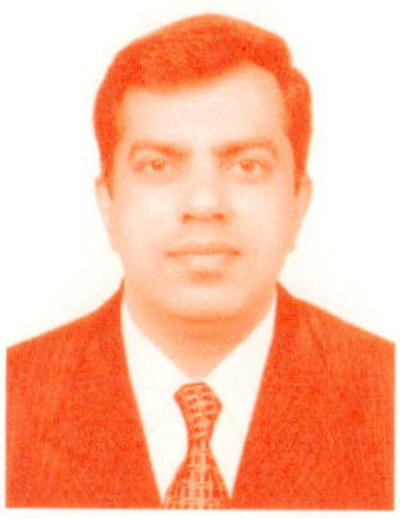
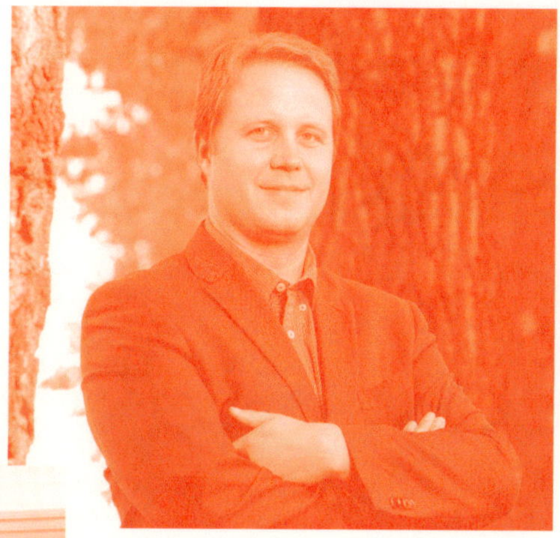
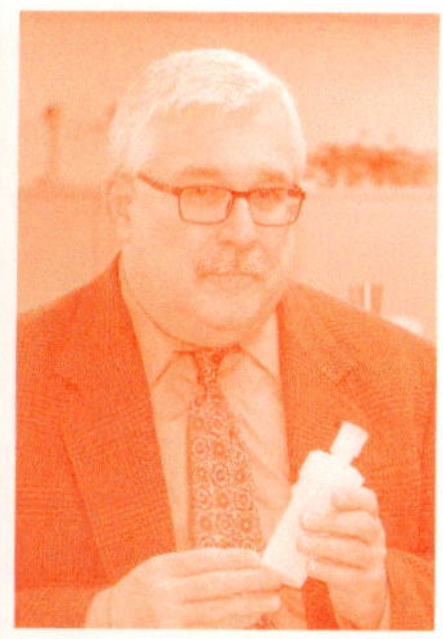
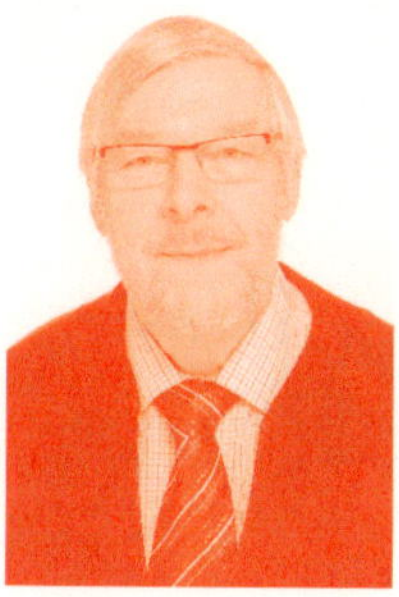
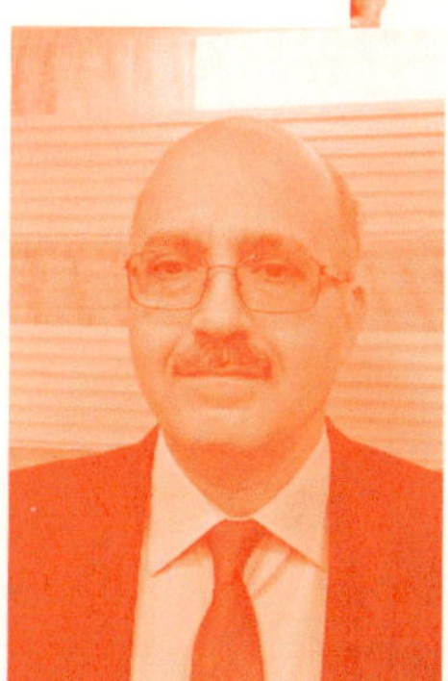
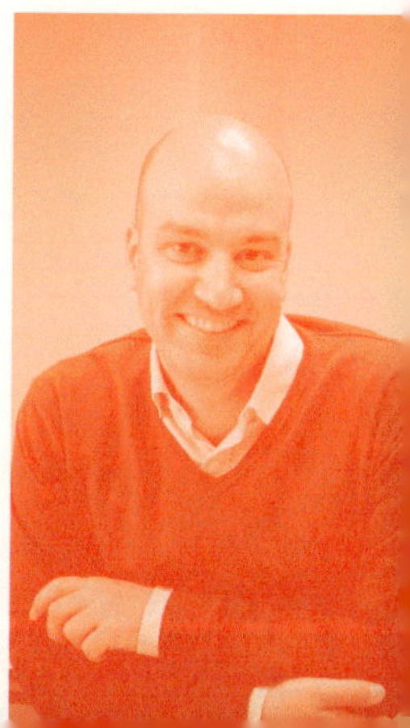
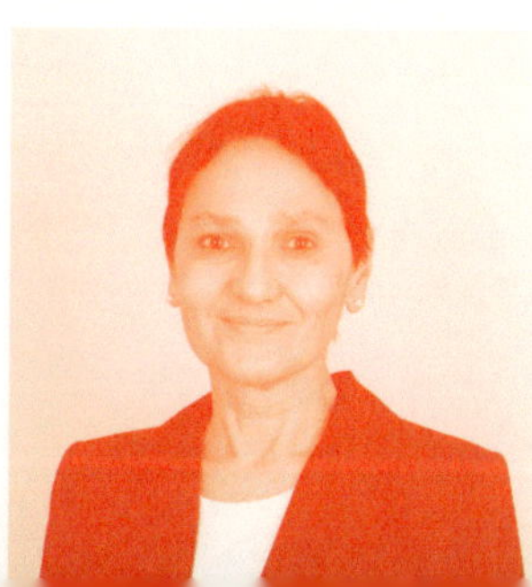

Selected Topics in Facial Nerve Disorders
http://dx.doi.org/10.5772/intechopen.73929
Edited by Isam Al-Zwaini and Mohammed Jalal Hussein

Contributors
Shu Yan Ng, Diego Rothschild, Hiroshi Moriyama, José Antonio A. Vega, Juan L. Cobo, Sonsoles Junquera, Antonio Sole-Magdalena, Juan Cobo, Isam Jaber Al-Zwaini

First published in London, United Kingdom, 2019 by IntechOpen
IntechOpen is the global imprint of INTECHOPEN LIMITED, registered in England and Wales, registration number: 11086078, The Shard, 25th floor, 32 London Bridge Street
London, SE19SG – United Kingdom
Printed in Croatia

British Library Cataloguing-in-Publication Data
A catalogue record for this book is available from the British Library

Additional hard copies can be obtained from orders@intechopen.com

Selected Topics in Facial Nerve Disorders
Edited by Isam Al-Zwaini and Mohammed Jalal Hussein
p. cm.
Print ISBN 978-1-83880-177-9
Online ISBN 978-1-83880-178-6

Meet the editors

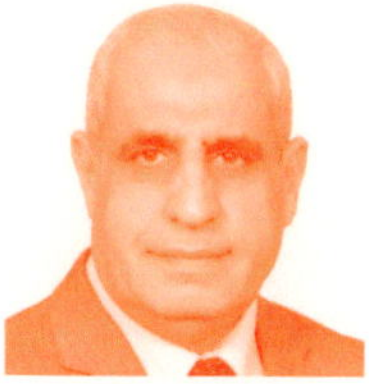

Prof. Isam Jaber Al-Zwaini was born on January 4, 1963, in Baghdad, Iraq. After graduating from Al-Mustansiryia College of Medicine in 1987, he worked as a house officer in different hospitals in Baghdad for 15 months, followed by military services for 3 years. He started his pediatric studies in 1991 and gained Fellowship of the Iraqi Commission for Medical Specializations in 1996. He worked as a lecturer in the Department of Pediatrics, Al-Anbar Medical College, from 1996 to 2001, where he upgraded to assistant professor in 2008. In 2007, he gained associate membership of the Royal College of Paediatrics and Child Health, UK. He has been the head of the Pediatric Department in Al-Anbar and Al-Kindy Medical College for many years. He has published more than 30 scientific papers in different pediatric fields, and his special interests are pediatric hematology, neurology, and nutrition.

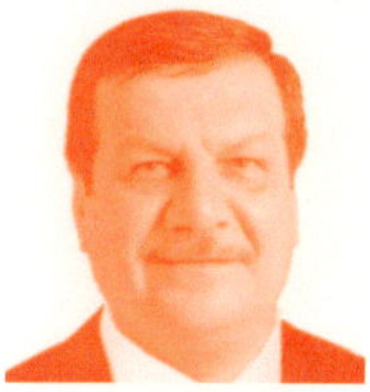

Prof. Mohammed Jalal Hussein was born on April 8, 1963, in Diayla, Iraq. After graduating from Al-Mustansiryia College of Medicine in 1987, he worked as a house officer in different hospitals in Baghdad for 15 months, followed by military services for 3 years. He started his pediatric studies in 1991 and gained Fellowship of the Iraqi Commission for Medical Specializations in 1995. He worked as a lecturer in the Department of Pediatrics, Tikrit Medical College, from 1996 to 1998, and has been working as a senior lecturer in Al-Kindy Medical College, Baghdad University, from 1998 until now. He upgraded to assistant professor in July 2000 and to professor in August 2008. In 2007, he gained associate membership of the Royal College of Paediatrics and Child Health, UK. He was the head of the pediatric department for many years and has been vice dean for Scientific Affairs in Al-Kindy Medical College since 2016. He has published more than 16 scientific papers in different pediatric fields and has a special interest in pediatric neurology.

Contents

Preface

The facial nerve (seventh cranial nerve) is the nerve of facial expression. It innervates all superficial muscles of the face and scalp, the contraction of which is responsible for all our numerous facial expressions like anger, pain, fear, smile, etc. Facial disfigurement resulting from facial nerve disorders can affect the physical, psychological, and emotional integrity of an individual. This might result in a social, occupational, and educational handicap. The facial nerve is one of the most common cranial nerves implicated by disorders. The content of this short book consists of three sections involving four chapters.

The first chapter is an introductory chapter by the editors, in which a brief account is given of facial nerve anatomy and common disorders involving the facial nerve like Bell's palsy, tumors, hemifacial spasm, and blepharospasm. Furthermore, we discuss common investigations used to diagnose facial nerve disorders and their clinical significance.

In the second chapter, Juan L. Cobo et al. discuss the role of proprioception in the regulation and coordination of facial musculature and diverse reflexes. The skeletal muscles contain an intrinsic mechanosensory system, the proprioceptive system, which provides information to the central nervous system about static and dynamic conditions of joints and muscles. In muscles, the proprioceptive system originates in specialized sensory organ-denominated muscle spindles. Nevertheless, facial muscles lack muscle spindles but facial proprioception plays key roles in the regulation and coordination of facial musculature and diverse reflexes. Facial proprioception, emanating from the facial muscles, plays key roles in facial expression and coordination of facial movement, regulation of the masticatory force in conjunction with jaw muscles, oromotor behaviors and nonverbal facial communication, as well as orofacial reflexes related to speech, swallowing, coughing, vomiting, or breathing. Moreover, proprioceptive acuity of the orofacial muscles has been found to be more accurate than the jaw. The chapter also discusses the multiple communications between the facial and trigeminal nerves and their role in conveying proprioceptive impulses via the branches of the trigeminal nerve to the central nervous system.

Professor Hiroshi Moriyama in the third chapter presents his original article about the treatment of facial nerve palsy based on genetic analysis of the facial muscles. He performed a genetic analysis of facial muscle specimens from Japanese patients with moderate (House-Brackmann facial nerve grading system III) and severe (House-Brackmann facial nerve grading system V) dysfunction due to Bell's palsy, and in rats after facial nerve resection (total paralysis). Microarray analysis of gene expression was performed using specimens from both the healthy and affected sides, and gene expressions were compared. The author defined changes in gene expression as a palsy/healthy side ratio >2.0 or <0.5. Changes of gene expression were observed; in particular, genes for muscle, neuron, and energy function showed changes with the severity of facial nerve palsy. This study may aid the development of new treatments and diagnostic/prognostic markers based on the severity of palsy.

In the fourth chapter, Dr. Ng Shu Yan et al. discuss the use of phototherapy for facial palsy. Various methods have been used to treat Bell's palsy, ranging from physical therapy to medications to decompression surgery. The standard treatment is currently a prescription of corticosteroids with antiviral agents. All these medical approaches yield mixed results and there is a need for an additional investigation on treatment options. Recent studies have shown that facial palsy responds positively to phototherapy treatment, in particular, the low-energy infrared laser. In this chapter, the authors review the current clinical application of phototherapy, representing a conservative and safe medical approach in the treatment of Bell's palsy. A literature review was also performed. The results of the included studies suggested that low-level laser therapy is a significant treatment modality for patients recovering from Bell's palsy. However, the risk of bias of the included studies was relatively high and further research could change the estimate of the effect of this treatment option.

Finally, I hope this short book with its interesting chapters will shed light on some of the remarkable aspects of the management of facial nerve disorders. I would like to thank all authors who contributed with their chapters and for their patience and cooperation throughout the processing of the book. In addition, I would like to express my sincere appreciation, deep thanks, and gratitude to the IntechOpen personnel, especially Ms. Kristina Kardum who offered me a great deal of help throughout the processing of this book.

Prof. Isam Jaber Al-Zwaini, PhD and Mohammed Jalal Hussein, PhD
Department of Pediatrics,
Al-Kindy Medical College,
University of Baghdad,
Baghdad, Iraq

Section 1

Introduction

Chapter 1

Introductory Chapter: Facial Nerve - An Overview

Isam Jaber Al-Zwaini and Mohammed Jalal Hussein

1. Introduction

The facial nerve (seventh cranial nerve—CNVII) is the nerve of facial expression. It innervates all superficial muscles of the face and scalp, the contraction of which is responsible for all our numerous facial expressions like anger, pain, fear, smile, etc. Facial disfigurement resulting from facial nerve disorders can affect the physical, psychological, and emotional integrity of an individual. This might result in social, occupational, and educational handicap. The facial nerve is one of the most common cranial nerves implicated by disorders. It is a mixed nerve, which carries motor, sensory, and parasympathetic fibers. The motor fiber-innervated muscles developed from second branchial arch, the sensory fibers transmit the special sense of taste, and the parasympathetic fibers supply the submandibular, sublingual, and lacrimal glands [1]. Embryologically speaking, it is formed very early within the acousticofacial complex from the second branchial arch [2]. Facial nerve consists of the juxtaposition of somatic and branchial elements of the cranial nerve nuclei, in particular, accounting for trigeminal and facial nerve anastomosis [3]. A wide variety of disorders can involve the facial nerve including congenital, traumatic, infectious, inflammatory, and neoplastic disorders.

2. Anatomy

The anatomy of the facial nerve is the most complex among other cranial nerves. It composed of approximately 10,000 neurons. Seven thousands of these fibers are myelinated and innervate the muscles of facial expression and the stapedial muscle. The other 3000 nerve fibers form the nervus intermedius with a secretary and somatosensory component. These include the afferent taste fiber from the chorda tympani nerve, the afferent taste fiber from the soft palate, the parasympathetic secretory innervation to sublingual, submandibular and lacrimal glands, and the cutaneous sensory component from afferent fibers originating from the skin of the auricle and postauricular areas [4]. The brain stem contains the *intraaxial segment*, which consists of the motor nucleus, superior salivary nucleus (parasympathetic), and nucleus of tractus solitarius (sensory). On the other hand, the *cisternal segment* consists of the motor root and nervus intermedius (nerve of Wrisberg), which emerge from the brain stem and pass into the internal auditory canal. These two segments merge at the internal auditory canal to form the *canalicular segment*. It runs in the internal auditory canal between the cochlea and vestibule of the inner ear to the geniculate ganglion forming the *labyrinthine segment*. From the geniculate ganglion, three nerves arise, the greater superficial petrosal nerve and lesser petrosal nerve carrying the parasympathetic fibers to the lacrimal and parotid gland

IntechOpen

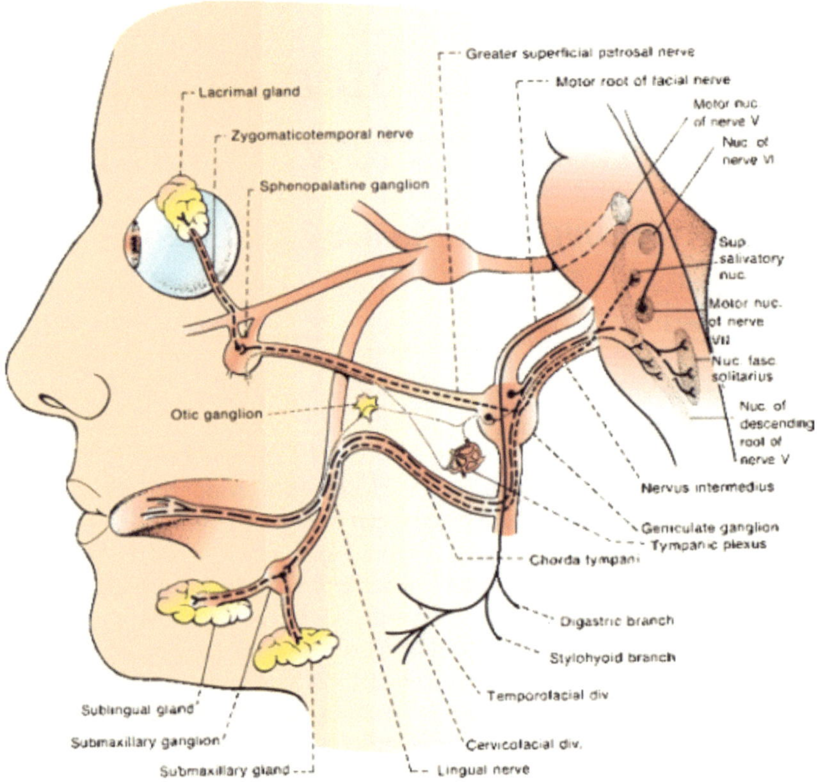

Figure 1.
The anatomy of the facial nerve. Adopted from the free domain: https://myneurosurg.com/cranial-anatomy/cranial-nerve-7-facial-nerve-and-its-pathology/.

and the external petrosal nerve supplying the sympathetic fibers to the middle meningeal artery. The nerve coursing from the geniculate ganglion to the pyramidal eminence forming the *tympanic segment*. From the pyramidal eminence, it passes down to the stylomastoid foramen forming the *mastoid segment* with branches to the stapedius muscle and chorda tympani. The *extracranial segment* started with emerging from the stylomastoid foramen, and it runs through the parotid gland giving rise to the superior temporozygomatic, inferior cervicofacial, temporal, zygomatic, buccal, mandibular, and cervical branches [5] (**Figure 1**).

Knowledge about the normal anatomy, vascular relationship, and the wide spectrum of the abnormalities is vital for the radiologist and neurologist in correctly diagnosing and managing facial nerve disorders.

3. Clinical disorders of facial nerve

3.1 Facial palsy

Bell's palsy is the idiopathic variety of facial nerve palsy where the patient has signs and symptoms of paralysis of facial muscles without known etiology. The etiologies that should be excluded in diagnosing Bell's palsy include intracranial and extracranial malignancies, infections, trauma, cerebrovascular accident, etc. Previously Bell's palsy was regarded as a diagnosis of exclusion, but in 1984, May et al. emphasized that Bell's palsy is a positive diagnosis based on specific clinical features [5]. The clinical features that may help to distinguish it from other causes of facial palsy include sudden onset of usually unilateral facial palsy with the absence of signs and symptoms of CNS, ear, and cerebellopontine angle disease. The annual incidence of Bell's palsy globally is estimated to be 11.5–53.3 per 100,000 in different population, and generally, the percentage is increasing as individuals get older [6–8], although some studies suggest that the highest incidence occurs among young and middle-aged individuals [9]. Bell's palsy thought to account for approximately 60–75% of cases of acute unilateral facial paralysis with the right side being affected in 63% of the time. It can also be recurrent with a reported recurrence range of 4–14% [10]. It affects both sexes equally but might affect women more than men in a certain age group. The lowest incidence is reported in persons younger than 10 years, and the highest incidence is in a person aged 70 years or older. Rarely it might occur bilaterally (0.3%), and positive family history is found in 4–14% of patients [11].

The pathophysiology of Bell's palsy remains unclear. Compression of the facial nerve while it course through facial canal, especially the narrow labyrinthine segment, is the most acceptable theory. The compression has been demonstrated in MRI scan with facial nerve enhancement [12]. Any inflammatory, demyelinating, and ischemic or compressive process in this area may impair the neural conduction. Viral infection is the most commonly accepted theory behind Bell's palsy, and the Herpes simplex virus is the most commonly implicated virus. Other viruses include Mumps virus, cytomegalovirus, and HIV. Other suggested theories include autoimmunity, mycoplasma infection, inflammation, microvascular disease such as diabetes mellitus, and many other mechanisms. It is apparent that none of these theories stands on a solid base.

Bell's palsy typically occurs suddenly, and the symptoms peak in less than 48 hours. The paralysis must include the upper and lower aspects of the face, otherwise, if it involves the lower portion of the face, a central cause (supranuclear), such as stroke, should be suspected. If the onset of the facial paralysis is insidious, associated with weakness of the contralateral side, or there is a preceding history of trauma or infection, other causes of facial paralysis must be strongly considered.

In addition to the sudden onset of unilateral upper and lower facial muscle paralysis, the patient may have hyperacusis, posterior auricular pain, otalgia, incomplete eye closure, excessive salivation, and taste disturbances. Many patients report numbness on the affected side. Whether this numbness is due to the involvement of trigeminal nerve or lack of movement of facial muscle is not clear. Ocular pain, epiphora or decreased tearing, and blurred vision are other possible associated symptoms.

On examination, in addition to demonstrate weakness and/or paralysis of the entire side of the face, we find a flattening of the nasolabial fold on the affected side, inability to elevate eyebrow, and distorted face when the patient asked to smile (**Figure 2**). The patient should be examined in details for full neurological examination, any skin lesion, ear or eye problem, and parotid diseases.

The goal of treatment of Bell's palsy is to improve the facial nerve function and to reduce neuronal damage. Steroids (prednisone) and antiviral therapy (acyclovir) are the recommended therapy by the American Academy of Neurology (AAN) and American Academy of Otolaryngology [13]. Additionally, a variety of non-pharmacological therapy is suggested for the treatment of Bell's palsy including physical therapy (facial exercises, neuromuscular training) and acupuncture. A variety of pharmacological and non-pharmacological treatments to protect the eyes of patient with Bell's palsy have been used. These include the use of topical ocular lubrication (with artificial tear during the day and lubricating ophthalmic ointment at night), occluding the eyelids by tape or patch, inducing ptosis by botulinum toxins, and many other procedures aiming to protect the patient's eye from drying, corneal abrasion, and corneal ulcers [14, 15].

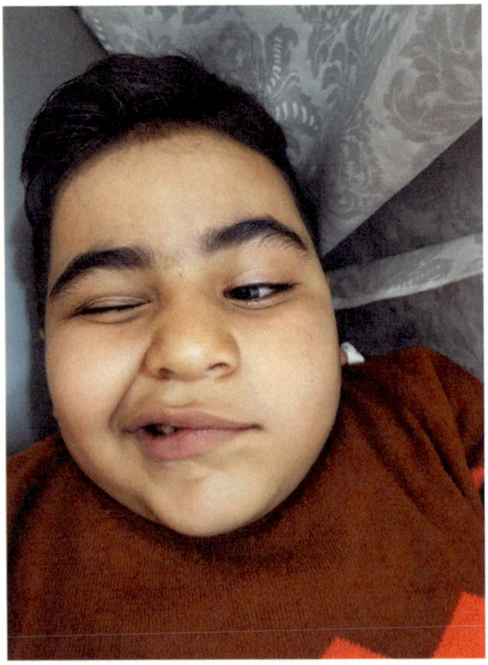

Figure 2.
Seven-year-old child with left facial palsy asked to smile (published with parent permission).

Surgical treatment of Bell's palsy with facial nerve decompression is also used, but it still carries a controversy, and it may be considered in patients with poor prognosis as predicted by facial nerve testing (EMG shows greater than 90% axonal degeneration within 3 weeks of the onset of paralysis) or complete persistent paralysis not responding to treatment [16, 17].

Other possible causes of facial palsy include congenital facial palsy (Möbius syndrome, hemifacial macrosomia), polyneuritis (Guillain-Barre syndrome, Ramsay-Hunt syndrome due to herpes zoster, autoimmune) malignancy (parotid tumors, brain tumor), trauma (temporal bone fracture, birth injury), sarcoidosis, infections (otitis media, cholesteatoma), and many other rare causes [18].

3.2 Tumors

Facial nerve tumors are rare and represent uncommon cause for facial palsy accounting for only 5–10% of all cases of facial nerve palsy [19]. Hearing defects and facial paresis are the most common presenting features. The most commonly identified tumor are schwannomas. Facial nerve schwannomas are benign tumors, which arise from Schwann cells. They mostly occur sporadically; some occur as a part of genetic syndromes as neurofibromatosis types 1 and 2. The facial nerve is the third common site for intracranial schwannomas. The patient usually presents with sudden onset or progressive facial weakness with or without conductive or sensorineural hearing loss, tinnitus, vertigo, facial pain, hemifacial spasm, facial palsy, and otalgia. Workup may involve detailed hearing test, MRI scan of the brain, and CT scan of the temporal bone. Other tumors involving the facial nerve include hemangiomas (accounting for 18% of facial nerve tumors and 0.7% of intratemporal bone tumors) [20], neurofibromas, and meningiomas. Most of these tumors present with facial palsy with or without hearing defects.

3.3 Hemifacial spasm (HFS)

It is a segmental myoclonus of muscles innervated by the facial nerve. Gowers first described it in 1884. It affects 11 per 100,000 of the population mostly in the fifth and sixth decade of life with a slight female predominance. The majority of cases are unilateral, although bilateral involvement might occur rarely in severe cases. It generally starts as brief clonic movements of the orbicularis oculi that spread over the years to other facial muscles (corrugator, frontalis, orbicularis oris, platysma, and zygomaticus), and it may become more sustained with time. Although it is a benign condition, it often leads to social embarrassment resulting in psychosocial stress and social withdrawal (**Figure 3**). HFS is characterized by progressive involuntary clonic or tonic movements of the muscle supplied by the facial nerve. It typically started in the orbicularis oculi muscle and progressively extends to involve the other facial muscle, involving the platysma muscle in severe cases. Most of the cases persist during sleep, and some patients report clicking sound in the ear, which presumed to be due to contraction of the stapedius muscle. In severe cases, impairment of vision might occur because of severe spasm of the orbicularis oculi muscle. The symptoms are usually exaggerated by psychological tension and speech. The main differential diagnosis of HFS includes blepharospasm (occur bilaterally symmetrically), oromandibular dystonia (sustained contraction of the lower part of the face, mouth, mandible and maxilla, tongue and pharynx), facial nerve tic (complex coordinated multifocal movement that switches between the right and left sides of the face), hemimasticatory spasm (painful contractions of the muscles of mastication), focal seizures, and synkinesias after facial nerve paralysis (activation of several muscles innervated by the facial nerve).

The underlying cause of hemifacial spasm in most cases is an ectatic or atypically aberrant blood vessel, which compresses the facial nerve at the place where it exits the brain stem. This area is the most susceptible part of the facial nerve to external stimuli since it ensheathed only by an arachnoidal membrane without the epineurium. Furthermore, this area represents the transition zone between central (oligodendroglial cells) and peripheral (Schwann cells) myelinations, and there is no connective tissue septa that traverse the individual fascicles. In the majority of cases, inferior posterior cerebellar artery or the inferior anterior cerebellar artery is the cause for vascular compression. Rarely, vertebral artery or a combination of these arteries is responsible for this compression. Very rarely, a vein might be the cause. HFS diagnosis is mainly clinically supported by investigations such as electromyography (EMG) and MRI. These investigations are useful also to exclude pathological changes in the cerebellopontine angle such as tumors or brain stem lesions. A high-resolution, T2-weighted sequence is particularly useful in demonstrating vascular compression.

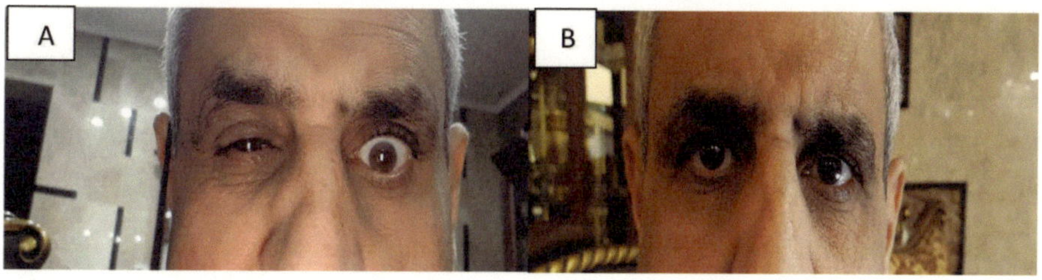

Figure 3.
The editor of this book is afflicted by right-sided HFS started at the age of 45; unfortunately, vascular decompression failed to resolve the problem. (A) Spasm of the right orbicularis oculi and right facial muscle and (B) spontaneous resolution of the spasm.

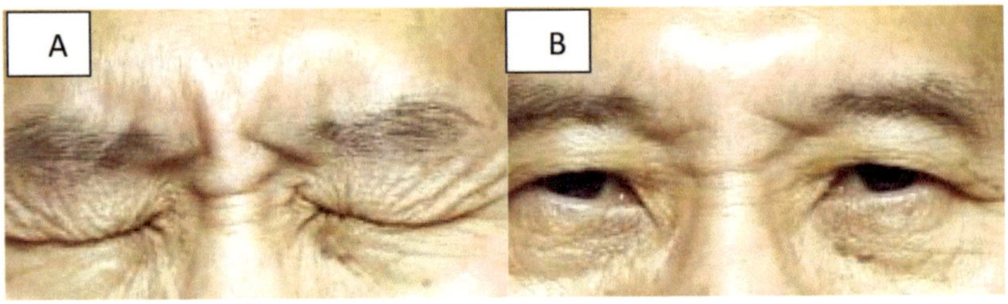

Figure 4.
(A) Patient with blepharospasm and (B) same patient after treatment.

The therapeutic options for HFS are variable ranging from simple applications of heat to pharmacological treatment (carbamazepine, clonazepam, baclofen, and gabapentin) and botulinum injections to microvascular decompression surgery. The response to medications, in general, is poor and not sustained and thus is devoted to milder cases. Botulinum toxin (BOTOX, BTX) became the standard treatment since its use in the early 1980s. It alleviates symptoms in 85–95% of patients. The major drawback is its temporary effects and the need to repeat its administration every 3–4 months [21–23]. The major advantages of BTX are that it is a noninvasive technique and can be done in an outpatient setting. The only curative therapeutic option is microvascular decompression of the facial nerve by placing a Teflon sponge between the vessel and the brain stem. Using an endoscopic technique makes the operation safe, but still, there is a risk of less than 1% of intraoperative life-threatening complications such as life-threatening hemorrhage or cerebellar or brain stem infarctions. Additionally, postoperative complications including temporary or permanent hearing impairment and permanent facial paralysis may occur in up to 8 and 0.9%, respectively [24].

3.4 Blepharospasm

It is the idiopathic progressive bilateral involuntary spasm of the orbicularis oculi and upper facial muscle (**Figure 4**). Involvement of the lower face by spasm is not uncommon, and the patient might be functionally blind as the eyes might be closed most of the day. The cause of the blepharospasm is thought to be central, yet the exact mechanism is not known. Treatment options include selective destruction of facial nerve branches that innervate the orbicularis oculi muscle, inducing paralysis of orbicularis oculi muscle by BOTOX, and pharmacological therapy by anticholinergics drug (Artane), benzodiazepine (clonazepam), GABAB receptor agonist (baclofen), anticonvulsant (levetiracetam), and many other drugs [25].

4. Investigations

In addition to a detailed history and clinical examination, investigations are an essential part of the workup of patients with facial nerve disorders. Still, there are controversies about the appropriate investigations that are needed for patients present with facial nerve disorders. The most commonly used investigations include:

4.1 Audiometry and brain stem auditory evoked response

These tests used to detect any associated hearing defect and diminished stapedial reflex (paresis of the stapedial branch of the facial nerve). Brain stem auditory evoked response (BAER) in particular is effective in detecting retrocochlear lesion. These tests are not used routinely unless there are multiple cranial nerve palsies [26, 27].

4.2 Full blood count

Facial paralysis is a recognized feature of leukemia relapses in both children and adult.

4.3 Imaging studies

Imaging studies play an important role in the evaluation of facial nerve disorder. MRI is especially helpful in recognizing brain stem pathology, and high-resolution CT scan is helpful in identifying bony abnormalities of the intratemporal facial nerve like congenital anomalies, trauma, and cholesteatoma. MRI is especially helpful in the detection of soft tissue abnormalities around facial nerve as in neoplasms, inflammatory processes, and hemifacial spasm. Recently, facial nerve ultrasound and diffuse tensor tractography (three-dimensional reconstruction of facial nerve using MRI) are used to identify cranial nerve fiber displacement by vestibular schwannomas [28, 29]. Contrast-enhanced MRI is helpful when the facial palsy cannot be definitively localized [30]. The patient's symptoms and the proposed differential diagnosis will determine the choice between these investigations.

4.4 Neurophysiological studies

Neurophysiological studies are of diagnostic and prognostic value, especially in chronic facial nerve problem. Most of these tests require the cooperation of patients. Examples of these tests include measurement of fibrillation potentials and recording of the blink reflex. The presence of fibrillation potentials, which is part of the electromyography, in the muscles implies the loss of muscle innervation, which indicates a significant axonal degeneration. Blink reflex tests, on the other hand, utilize the polysynaptic nature of this reflex. Trigeminal nerve carries a unilateral stimuli (electric stimulation of the supraorbital nerve or a puff of air on the cornea), producing an early ipsilateral facial motor response followed by a bilateral late response. Absence or delay in the late response can be used to assess facial innervation [31].

Author details

Isam Jaber Al-Zwaini* and Mohammed Jalal Hussein
Department of Pediatrics, Al-Kindy Medical College, University of Baghdad, Baghdad, Iraq

*Address all correspondence to: ejkzwaini@yahoo.com

References

[1] Mortazavi MM, Latif B, Verma K, et al. The fallopian canal: A comprehensive review and proposal of a new classification. Child's Nervous System. 2014;**30**(3):387-395

[2] Toulgoat F, Sarrazin JL, Benoudib F, Pereon Y, Auffray-Calvier E, Daumas-Duport B, et al. Facial nerve: From anatomy to pathology. Diagnostic and Interventional Imaging. 2013;**94**:1033-1042

[3] Lacombe H. Anatomie fonctionnelle du nerf facial. Neurochirurgie 2009;**55**(2):113-9

[4] Available from: https://emedicine.medscape.com/article/835286-overview

[5] Ho M-L, Juliano A, Eisenberg RL, Moonis G. Anatomy and pathology of the facial nerve. AJR. 2015;**204**:W612-W619

[6] Rowhani-Rahbar A, Baxter R, Rasgon B, Ray P, Black S, Klein JO, et al. Epidemiologic and clinical features of Bell's palsy among children in northern California. Neuroepidemiology. 2012;**38**:252-258. DOI: 10.1159/000338303

[7] Brandenburg NA, Annegers JF. Incidence and risk factors for Bell's palsy in Laredo, Texas: 1974-1982. Neuroepidemiology. 1993;**12**:313-325

[8] Katusic SK, Beard CM, Wiederholt WC, Bergstralh EJ, Kurland LT. Incidence, clinical features, and prognosis in Bell's palsy, Rochester, Minnesota, 1968-1982. Annals of Neurology. 1986;**20**:622-627

[9] De Diego JI, Prim MP, Madero R, Gavilàn J. Seasonal patterns of idiopathic facial paralysis: A 16-year study. Otolaryngology and Head and Neck Surgery. 1999;**120**:269-271. DOI: 10.1016/S0194-5998(99)70418-3

[10] Peitersen E. Bell's palsy: The spontaneous course of 2,500 peripheral facial nerve palsies of different etiologies. Acta Oto-Laryngologica. Supplementum. 2002;**549**:4-30

[11] Girbau A, Perez N, Fernandez N, Lorente Caparrós M, Torra Parra L, Solà Ruano R, et al. Familial Bell's palsy: A case report. Annals of Physical and Rehabilitation Medicine. 2018;**61**:e262

[12] Seok JI, Lee DK, Kim KJ. The usefulness of clinical findings in localising lesions in Bell's palsy: Comparison with MRI. Journal of Neurology, Neurosurgery, and Psychiatry. 2008;**79**(4):418-420

[13] Grogan PM, Gronseth GS. Practice parameter: Steroids, acyclovir, and surgery for Bell's palsy (an evidence-based review): Report of the quality standards Subcommittee of the American Academy of Neurology. Neurology. 2001;**56**(7):830-836

[14] Holland NJ, Weiner GM. Recent developments in Bell's palsy. BMJ. 2004;**329**(7465):553-557

[15] Seiff SR, Chang J. Management of ophthalmic complications of facial nerve palsy. Otolaryngologic Clinics of North America. 1992;**25**(3):669-690

[16] Gilden DH. Clinical practice. Bell's palsy. The New England Journal of Medicine. 2004;**351**(13):1323-1331

[17] Julian GG, Hoffmann JF, Shelton C. Surgical rehabilitation of facial nerve paralysis. Otolaryngologic Clinics of North America. 1997;**30**(5):701-726

[18] Mavrikakis L. Facial nerve palsy: Anatomy, etiology, evaluation, and management. Orbit. 2008;**27**:466-474

[19] Jackson CG, Glasscock ME, Hughes F, et al. Facial paralysis of neoplastic origin, diagnosis and management. Laryngoscope. 1980;**90**:1581-1595

[20] Zhi-Yao S, Li J. Facial nerve hemangiomas: A review. Journal of Otology. 2012;7(1):28-30

[21] Wang A, Jankovic J. Hemifacial spasm: Clinical findings and treatment. Muscle & Nerve. 1998;**21**:1740-1747

[22] Barker FG 2nd, Jannetta PJ, Bissonette DJ, Shields PT, Larkins MV, Jho HD. Microvascular decompression for hemifacial spasm. Journal of Neurosurgery. 1995;**82**:201-210

[23] Simpson DM, Blitzer A, Brashear A, et al. Therapeutics and technology assessment Subcommittee of the American Academy of Neurology. Assessment: Botulinum neurotoxin for the treatment of movement disorders (an evidence-based review): Report of the therapeutics and technology assessment Subcommittee of the American Academy of neurology. Neurology. 2008;**70**:1699-1706

[24] Rosenstengel C, Matthes M, Baldauf J, Fleck S, Schroeder H. Hemifacial spasm—Conservative and surgical treatment options. Deutsches Ärzteblatt International. 2012;**109**(41):667-673. DOI: 10.3238/arztebl.2012.0667

[25] Anderson RL, Patel BC, Holds JB, Jordan DR. Blepharospasm: Past, present, and future. Ophthalmic Plastic and Reconstructive Surgery. 1998;**14**(5):305-317

[26] Hendrix RA, Melnick W. Auditory brain stem response and audiologic tests in idiopathic facial nerve paralysis. Otolaryngology and Head and Neck Surgery. 1983;**91**(6):686-690

[27] Shanon E, Himelfarb MZ, Zikk D. Measurement of auditory brain stem potentials in Bell's palsy. The Laryngoscope. 1985;**95**(2):206-209

[28] Lo YL, Fook-Chong S, Leoh TH, et al. High-resolution ultrasound in the evaluation and prognosis of Bell's palsy. European Journal of Neurology. 2010;**17**(6):885-889

[29] Taoka T, Hirabayashi H, Nakagawa H, et al. Displacement of the facial nerve course by vestibular schwannoma: Preoperative visualization using diffusion tensor tractography. Journal of Magnetic Resonance Imaging. 2006;**24**(5):1005-1010

[30] Gupta S, Mends F, Hagiwara M, Fatterpekar G, Roehm PC. Imaging the facial nerve: A contemporary review. Radiology Research and Practice. 2013;**2013**:248039

[31] Riordan M. Investigation and treatment of facial paralysis. Archives of Disease in Childhood. 2001;**84**:286-287

Section 2

Facial Nerve and Proprioception

Chapter 2

The Proprioception in the Muscles Supplied by the Facial Nerve

Juan L. Cobo, Antonio Solé-Magdalena, Sonsoles Junquera, Teresa Cobo, José Antonio Vega and Juan Cobo

Abstract

Proprioception is a quality of somatosensibility that informs the central nervous system about the static and dynamics of muscles and joints. In muscles, the proprioceptive originates in the specialized sensory-organ-denominated muscle spindles. Nevertheless, facial muscles lack muscle spindles, but the facial proprioception plays key roles in the regulation and coordination of facial musculature and diverse reflexes. At the basis of these functional characteristics are the multiple communications between the facial and the trigeminal nerves, and neuroanatomical studies have demonstrated that facial proprioceptive impulses are conveyed via branches of the trigeminal nerve to the central nervous system. Substituting muscle spindles facial muscles contain other kinds of proprioceptors of variable morphology that display immunoreactivity for some putative mechanoproteins known to participate in proprioception (acid-sensing ion channel 2, transient receptor potential vanilloid 4, and Piezo2).

Keywords: facial muscles, facial nerve, trigemino-facial communications, proprioception, innervation, mechanoproteins

1. Introduction

The facial and trigeminal nerves are cranial nerves (CN) responsible for the motor and sensory innervation of the craniocephalic muscles and skin of the face, respectively. All the classic texts of Human Anatomy describe with detail the origin, branching patterns and anatomical variants of both trigeminal (CNV) and facial (CNVII) nerves, and it can be think that little new can be say of these nerves. Nevertheless, nothing so far from the reality since complexes communications exists between them. In fact, almost all the terminal branches of CNVII receive numerous communications from branches of CNV whose fibers accompany those of CNVII until muscles form sensorimotor units. Therefore, CNVII, at least at the terminal level, is mixed and no purely motor. Although studies in humans do not exist, the data collected from animal models indicate that the nerve fiber interchange is always from CNV to CNVII and not on the contrary [1].

The skeletal muscles contain an intrinsic mechanosensory system, the proprioceptive system, which provides information to the central nervous system about static and dynamic conditions of joints and muscles [2, 3]. The proprioceptive inputs originate in specialized sensory organs (proprioceptors) present in muscles (muscle spindles [4, 5]), tendons (Golgi's tendon organs [6]), and joint capsules

(Ruffini-like sensory corpuscles, Pacinian corpuscles, and free nerve endings [7]). Furthermore, it has been proposed that some kinds of cutaneous mechanoreceptors can also work as proprioceptors, but their physiological properties suggest they are not the alternative to muscle spindles [8–11].

Proprioception is a part of mechanosensation that involves all skeletal muscles, including the craniocephalic ones. But while muscles innervated by CNV contain typical proprioceptors [12, 13], i.e., muscle spindles, in those innervated by CNVII, they are absent (see [14]). However, facial proprioception, emanated from the facial muscles, plays key roles in facial expression and coordination of facial movement, regulation of the masticatory force in conjunction with jaw muscles, oromotor behaviors, and nonverbal facial communication, as well as in orofacial reflexes related to speech, swallowing, coughing, vomitting, or breathing [14]. Moreover, proprioceptive acuity of the orofacial muscles has been found to be more accurate than the jaw [15].

Some decades ago, Baumel [16] suggested that proprioceptive impulses from facial muscles are conveyed to the central nervous system via different branches of CNV throughout multiple communications with the branches of CNVII, and actually it is accepted that the proprioception of the craniocephalic muscles depends on CNV [14, 17].

All together, the above data suggest complex anatomical and functional intercommunication between CNV and CNVII which are of capital importance to understand the clinic of these nerves.

Here we have reviewed the literature of the connections between CNV and CNVII as well as the actual knowledge about facial proprioception. Moreover we added our experience in those fields with results from anatomical dissections and analyzed the proprioceptors present in facial muscles.

2. An overview of CNV and CNVII

CNV and CNVII are both mixed cranial nerves that carry motor and sensory fibers responsible for both the sensory and motor innervation of the face, respectively. Moreover, CNVII and some branches of CNV contain preganglionic and postganglionic parasympathetic nerve fibers [18, 19].

2.1 Trigeminal nerve: CNV

CNV is responsible for the sensory innervation of the face, both skin and mucosae, and the motor innervation of the craniocephalic muscles originated from the first pharyngeal arch. It apparently originates by two roots at the midlateral surface of pons that reach the Gasser's ganglion where it divides into three branches denominated ophthalmic (sensory CNV1), maxillary (sensory CNV2), and mandibular (mixed CNV3). The soma of the trigeminal somatosensory neurons is localized in the trigeminal ganglion (Gasser's ganglion), whereas the proprioceptive ones, i.e., those innervating craniofacial muscles, are localized in the nucleus mesencaphalicus nervi trigemini [18, 19].

2.2 Facial nerve—CNVII

CNVII is responsible for the innervation and control of the movements of all the craniofacial muscles, with exceptions of jaw muscles. Moreover, it innervates some muscles in the neck and middle ear. The sensory territory of CNVII includes the anterior two-thirds of the tongue, a part of the outer ear skin, and the so-called Ramsey-Hunt's zone. CNVII originates at the pontocerebellar angle by two roots: the largest root motor and the smaller root sensitive (the so-called intermediate Wrisberg's nerve; *N. intermedius*). Both roots enter the temporal bone, continue through the facial canal and fuse, and finally emerge at the foramen stylomastoideum. Within the parotid gland, CNVII bifurcates into two primary trunks: larger temporo-facial and a smaller cervicofacial trunk. The two primary trunks form the parotid plexus and thus form connections along six distinctive anastomotic types in 44% of the cases [20]. Thereafter, from the parotid plexus originates five major branches (with wide variations): temporal (r. temporales), the zygomatic (r. zygomatici), the buccal (r. buccales), mandibular (*R. marginalis* mandibularis), and the cervical (r. cervicales) [18, 19, 21–23].

Nevertheless, the peripheral branching and intercommunication of the facial branches were highly variable [24]. In our experience on 10 hemi heads we observed a different pattern of facial nerve branching between subjects and between right and left sides from the same subject. According to the Davis et al. classification [25] of the facial nerve based on the patterns of facial nerve branching, we observed that type II (6/10) predominates, followed by type IV (3/10) and type V (1/10). But independently of the type communicating branches between the different the main terminal branches of CNVII were found (**Figure 1**; [26]).

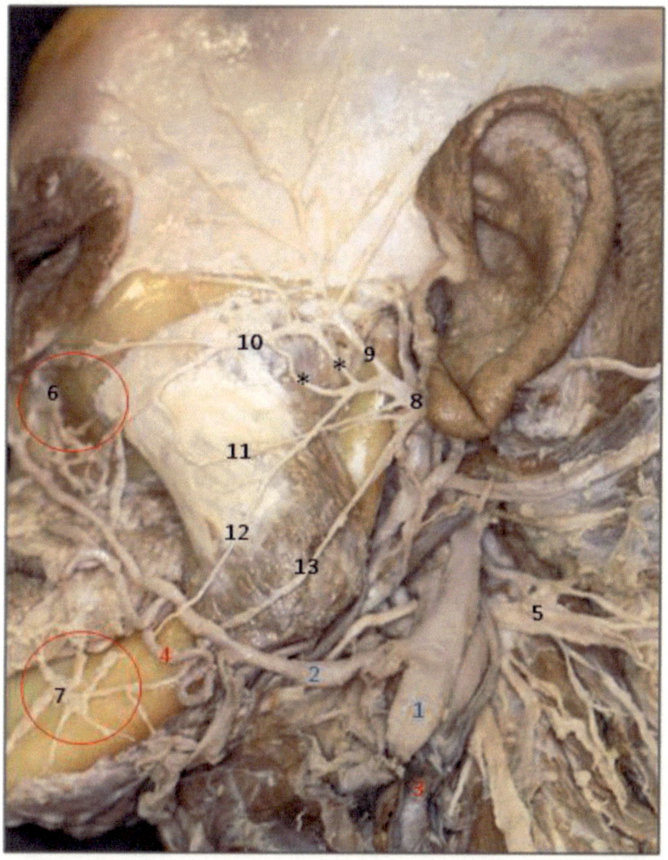

Figure 1.
*Cadaveric dissection of the left facial nerve in the hemi-head of a male, 66 years old. The facial nerve branched within the parotid gland (removed) into five branches largely connected between them at the initial segments. 1, external jugular vein; 2, facial vein; 3, external carotid artery; 4, facial artery; 5, CN XI; 6, infraorbital branch of CNV2; 7, mental nerve CNV3; 8, CN VII; 9, temporal branches of CNVII; 10, zygomatic branch of CNVII; 11, buccal branches of CNVII; 12, mandibular branches of CNVII; 13, cervical branches of CNVII; *, connections between primary facial trunks. This image was obtained from our own dissections and was carried out at the area of anatomy and human embryology, Department of Morphology and Cell Biology, University of Oviedo, Spain. Similar image from the same dissection was published previously by Cobo et al. [42].*

In addition to the main primary branches mentioned above, in some cases an aberrant branch arose from the main trunk before bifurcation and numerous anatomical variants. Moreover connections between the facial nerve branches have been described [27, 28].

The somatosensory and gustative peripheral neurons of CNVII are localized in the ganglion geniculatum, and their central branch terminates in the nucleus tractus solitarius of the brainstem. The motor axons originate from neurons located in nucleus nervi facialis. CNVII innervates the derivatives of the second branchial arch of the embryos, including facial muscles.

3. Communications between CNV and CNVII

CNVII exhibits a highly variable and complicated branching pattern and forms communications with several other cranial nerves, especially with branches of all three divisions of CNV [20, 29–42].

The revision about trigemino-facial communications carried out by Hwang et al. [33] shows in cadaveric studies the highest frequency of communication of CNVII is with CNV2 (95.0% ± 8.0%), followed by CNV3 (76.7% ± 38.5%) and CNV1 (33.8% ± 19.5%). However using nerve impregnation methods, the communications reach 100% for CNV2 and CNV3 and 85.7% for CNV1 [39]. Interestingly, communication between the infraorbital nerve and the different branches of CNVII is regularly found just below the infraorbital foramen, forming the infraorbital plexus [30, 36, 42]. Another regular connection is between the mental nerve of CNV3 and the mandibular branch of the facial nerve [42]. On the other hand, CNVII can receive proprioceptive information from the cervical nerves which are frequency communicated (65.2 ± 43.5%; [33]), as well as with the auriculotemporal nerve [34, 43].

Interestingly, although independent of CNV, the connection between the great auricular nerve (composed of branches of spinal nerves C2 and C3) and CNVII trunk has been regularly observed (100%) [44], which probably serves the platysma colli. Functionally, these communications consistently innervated some of the muscles of upper facial expression and presumably are also responsible of their proprioception. Anastomoses in the neck between the sensory transverse cervical nerve (C2 and C3) and the cervical branch of the facial nerve are common, but communications with more superior branches of the facial nerve are rare [45].

4. Sensory innervation of the facial muscles

All the craniofacial muscles except the jaw ones are innervated by CNVII. To understand the proprioceptive innervation of the facial muscles, it is necessary to know as they are innervated by CNVII branches and as terminal segments of the facial nerves contain sensory fibers coming from CNV that provide these muscles with proprioceptive fibers, although individual differences may exist. The innervation of the facial muscles is summarized in **Figure 2** [46].

The facial muscles are devoid of proprioceptors, and therefore facial movements lack a conventional proprioceptive feedback system, which may be only in part vicariate by cutaneous afferents [10, 47]. Therefore, a putative facial proprioceptive system, if present, must be represented by other structures not identified yet.

4.1 Proprioceptors in facial muscles

In the middle of the last century, Kadanoff [48] investigated the innervation of the human facial muscles using silver impregnation techniques and observed

Trigeminal nerve branches	Facial nerve branches	Muscles
auriculotemporal great auricular	Facial trunks: temporo--facial Cervico-facial	
zygomatictemporal supraorbital auriculotemporal	Temporal branch	fontalis procerus depressor supercilii corrugator supercilii orbicularis oculi
supraorbital supratroclear buccinators buccal zygomaticofacial auriculotemporal	Zygomatic branch	orbicularis oculi zygomaticus major zygomaticus minor levator labii superioris aleque nasi levator anguli oris
nfratrochlear infraorbital buccal mental bucinator zygomaticofacial auriculotemporal	Buccal branch	orbicularis oculi zygomaticus major zygomaticus minor levator labii superioris aleque nasi levator anguli oris buccinators risorius
buccinator mental	Mandibular branch	orbicularis oris depressor anguli oris depressor labii inferioris mentalis
	Cervical branch	platysma

Figure 2.
Schematic presentation of the communications between CNV branches and the main divisions of CNVII to provide sensory innervation to the facial muscles. Data are based on the literature cited in the manuscript.

numerous and varied morphotypes of sensory nerve endings in the facial muscles, especially in the perioral ones. Nevertheless, as far as we know, no typical muscle spindles have been found in the human facial muscles [49–53] More recently, Cobo et al. [54] have not found any morphological or immunohistochemical evidence for the presence of muscle spindles in two facial muscles, while they were regularly present in the masseter muscle. Conversely, one muscle spindle was found in the muscle orbicularis oculi in one pediatric specimen [55], and abundant muscle spindles have been found in the platysma colli [56].

Recently we have conducted a research focused to identify proprioceptors, other than muscle spindles, in human facial muscles [26, 54]. The identification of putative sensory receptors in the facial muscles was based on the following criteria: independence of the nerve trajectory, be placed in close relation to muscle fibers, display a morphologically differentiated aspect, and display immunoreactivity for any putative mechanoprotein (**Figure 3**).

In no case were typical muscle spindles found, whereas in the masseter muscle (used as a control) typical muscle spindles were found (**Figure 4**). In agreement with the above premises, we identified capsulated and non-capsulated corpuscle-like structures of variable size and shape containing numerous axon profiles complexly arranged, which resembled elongated or round Ruffini-like corpuscles (**Figure 5**).

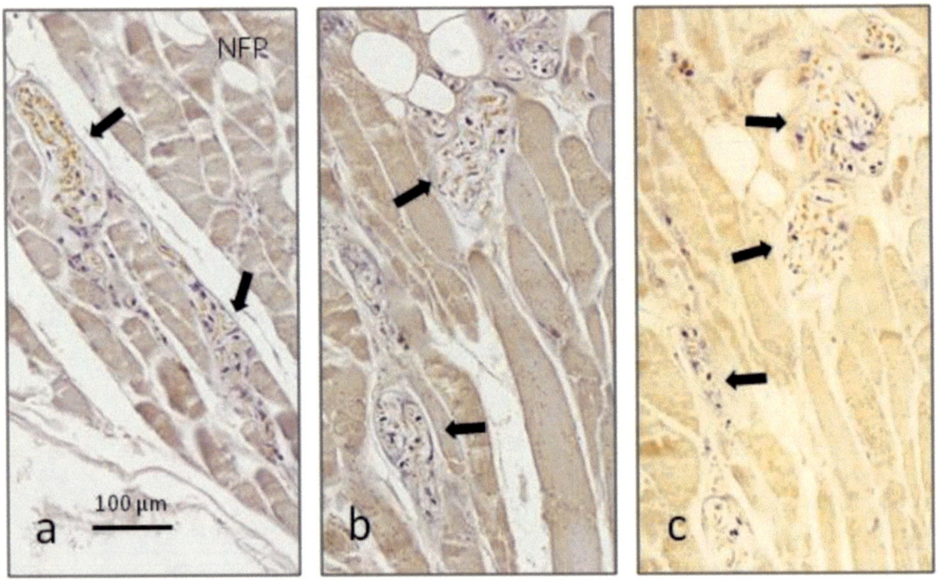

Figure 3.
Sensory nerve formations in the facial muscles (arrows) displaying immunoreactivity for the axonal marker neurofilament protein (NFP). a, buccal muscle; b, zygomaticus major muscle; c, orbicularis oris muscle.

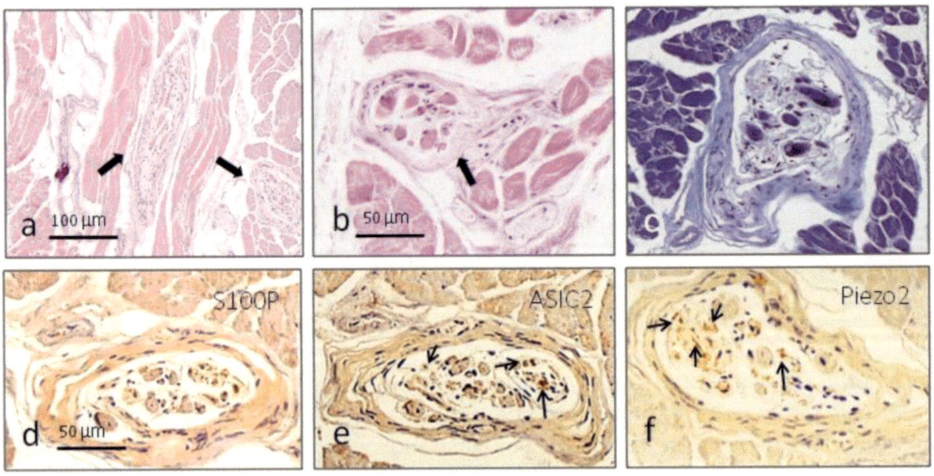

Figure 4.
Longitudinal (a) and cross (b,c) sections of two typical muscle spindles in the human masseter muscle (arrows) containing a variable number of intrafusal muscle fibers. Nerve fibers supplying them display immunoreactivity for Schwann cells markers like S100 protein (d) and the putative mechanoproteins ASIC2 (e, arrows) and Piezo2 (f, arrows).

Given the morphologic heterogeneity of the corpuscle-like structures that fulfill the preestablished criteria we attempt to classify them into three types: type I, capsulated by a thin capsule and the glial cells variably arranged and showing different morphologies (**Figure 6a**); type II, partially capsulated (the capsule being continuous with the perimysium), with variable morphology, and in most of the cases the direction of the long axis was parallel to the one of muscular fibers (**Figure 6b**); and type III, non-capsulated and both the axon and Schwann-like cells are variably arranged (**Figure 6c**).

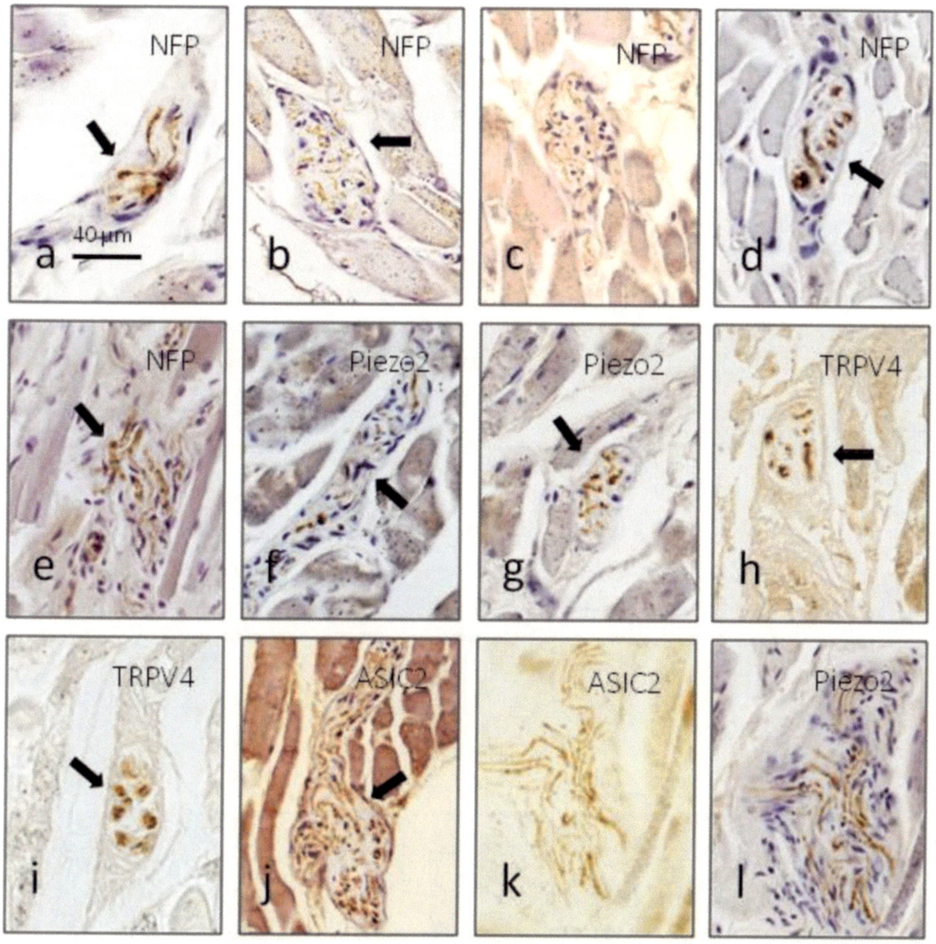

Figure 5.
Different morphotypes of corpuscle-like structures (arrows) identified immunohistochemically using axonal markers (a–e) and putative mechanoproteins (f–l). In serial sections (k and l), apparent co-localization of two mechanoproteins in the axon is observed.

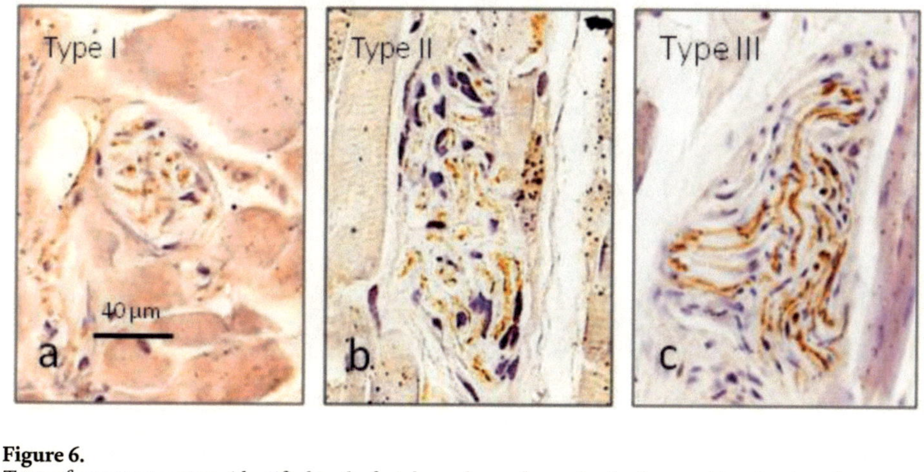

Figure 6.
Types of sensory structures identified in the facial muscles as observed using immunohistochemistry for neurofilament proteins.

Muscle	Type I	Type II	Type III	Fibers*
M. corrugator supercilii + M. depresor supercilii	1	3	7	Yes
M. orbicularis oculi pars palpebralis pars orbitalis	3	11	9	Yes
M. orbicularis oris pars marginalis pars labialis	5	19	12	Yes
M. zygomaticus major	1	4	4	Yes
M. zygomaticus minor	1	2	0	Yes
M. buccinator	19	28	10	Yes
M. depressor labii inferioris + mentalis	0	8	2	

**Isolated nerve fibers displaying immunoreactivity for any of the mechanoproteins investigated.*

Table 1.
Relative density of proprioceptors in human facial muscles. Counts were made on 10 sections separated de 200 μm between them.

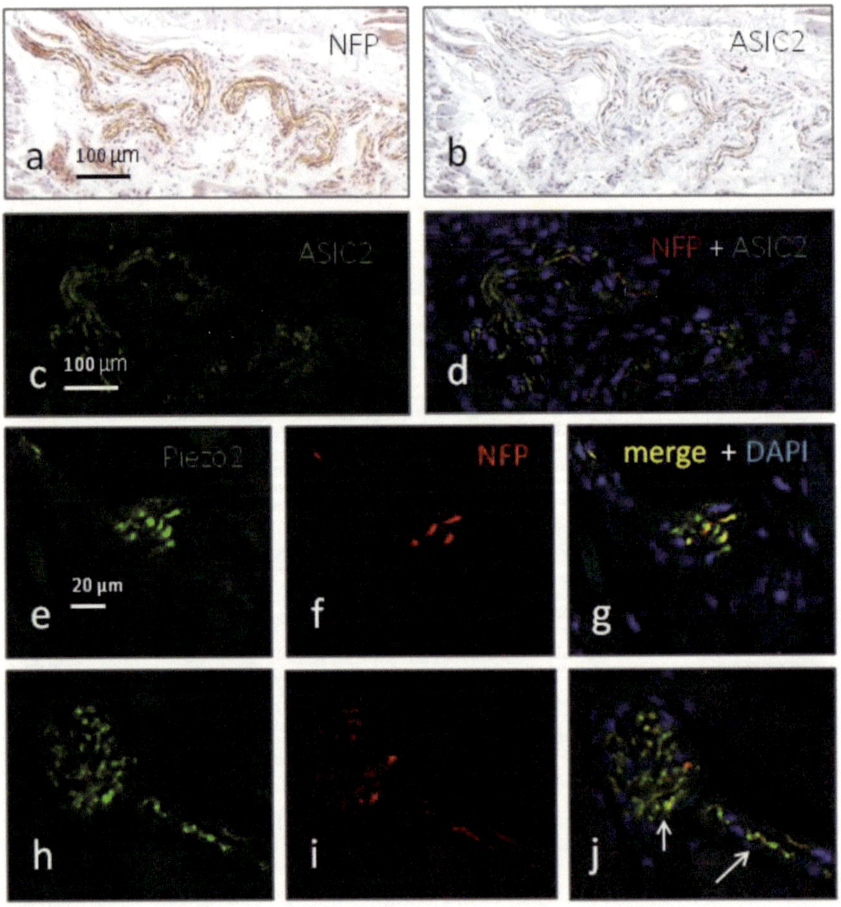

Figure 7.
Serial sections processed for the detection of neurofilament protein (NFP) and ASIC2 showing that a subpopulation of the axons in nerves supplying the facial nerves contains mechanoproteins (a,b). Nerves and capsulated corpuscle-like structures (types I and II) immunostained with anti-ASIC2 (c) or anti-Piezo2 (e,h) antibodies conjugated with Alexa fluor 488 (green fluorescence) and with anti-NFP antibody conjugated with CyTM3 (red fluorescence). The localization of the putative mechanoproteins ASIC2 and Piezo2 in the large axons was evident while it was not so clear in the thick axons.

On the other hand, the relative density of proprioceptors in the facial muscles varied from one to another (**Table 1**), the greater density being observed in the buccinator and orbicularis oris muscles, and the type II of proprioceptors being the predominating morphotype.

All sensory modalities involve different ion channels, and at the basis of mechanosensibility are mechanically gated membrane ion channels [5, 57]. At present acid-sensing ion channel 2 (ASIC2), transient receptor potential vanilloid 4 (TRPV4), and Piezo2 have been detected in muscle spindles and are strong candidates to initiate the mechanotransduction in proprioceptors [57–61]. In the studies, we have carried out [54] regularly found is immunoreactivity for ASIC2, TRPV4, and Piezo2 in the axon of types I, II, and III facial sensory corpuscles, thus confirming that these structures may serve as proprioceptors (**Figure 5f-l**). In serial sections (**Figure 7a** and **b**) with our use of double immunofluorescence and laser confocal microscopy (**Figure 7c-j**), it was observed that a subpopulation of nerve fibers displays immunoreactivity for the putative mechanoproteins and that these proteins are localized in the axon of the sensory structures within the facial muscles, thus confirming their proprioceptive function.

5. Concluding remarks

The facial muscles are richly innervated by sensory fibers that form at the periphery of different types of sensory structures of variable complexity which express putative mechanoproteins and therefore can be regarded as proprioceptors. Conversely facial muscles lack typical muscles spindles. Presumably, the sensory fibers forming the facial muscle proprioceptors originate in CNV. Because of the high variability in the pattern of branching and distribution of CNVII as well as of their communications with other CNs especially CNV, a correct knowledge of the anatomy of those nerves to preserve it when performing surgical or medical procedures in the face is necessary since a disruption of these connections might alter facial muscle proprioception. These communications have clinical significance for recovery of damaged facial expression muscles, treatment of hemifacial spasm, and surgical procedures for facial reconstruction and neck dissection.

Author details

Juan L. Cobo[1,2], Antonio Solé-Magdalena[1,3], Sonsoles Junquera[4], Teresa Cobo[5,6], José Antonio Vega[1,7]* and Juan Cobo[5,6]

1 Departamento de Morfología y Biología Celular, Grupo SINPOS, Universidad de Oviedo, Spain

2 Servicio de Cirugía Máxilo-Facial, Hospital Universitario Central de Asturias, Oviedo, Spain

3 Servicio de Hematología, Hospital Universitario Central de Asturias, Oviedo, Spain

4 Servicio de Radiologia, Hospital Universitario, Santiago de Compostela, Spain

5 Departamento de Cirugía y Especialidades Médico-Quirúrgicas, Universiada de Oviedo, Spain

6 Instituto Asturiano de Odontología, Oviedo, Spain

7 Facultad de Ciencias de la Salud, Universid Autónoma de Chile, Temunco, Chile

*Address all correspondence to: javega@uniovi.es

References

[1] Bowden RE, Mahran ZY. Experimental and histological studies of the extrapetrous portion of the facial nerve and its communications with the trigeminal nerve in the rabbit. Journal of Anatomy. 1960;**94**:375-386

[2] Dijkerman HC, de Haan EH. Somatosensory processes subserving perception and action. The Behavioral and Brain Sciences. 2007;**30**:189-201

[3] Butler AA, Héroux ME. Gandevia SC. Body ownership and a new proprioceptive role for muscle spindles. Acta Physiologica (Oxford, England). 2016;**220**:19-27

[4] Banks RW. The innervation of the muscle spindle: A personal history. Journal of Anatomy. 2015;**227**:115-135

[5] Bewick GS, Banks RW. Mechanotransduction in the muscle spindle. Pflügers Archiv. 2015;**467**:175-190

[6] Ackermann PW, Salo P, Hart DA. Tendon innervation. Advances in Experimental Medicine and Biology. 2016;**920**:35-51

[7] Heppelmann B. Anatomy and histology of joint innervation. Journal of the Peripheral Nervous System. 1997;**2**:5-16

[8] Collins DF, Refshauge KM, Todd G, Gandevia SC. Cutaneous receptors contribute to kinesthesia at the index finger, elbow, and knee. Journal of Neurophysiology. 2005;**94**:1699-1706

[9] Macefield VG. Physiological characteristics of low-threshold mechanoreceptors in joints, muscle and skin in human subjects. Clinical and Experimental Pharmacology & Physiology. 2005;**32**:135-144

[10] Andreatta RD, Barlow SM. Somatosensory gating is dependent on the rate of force recruitment in the human orofacial system. Journal of Speech, Language, and Hearing Research. 2009;**52**:1566-1578

[11] Proske U, Gandevia SC. The proprioceptive senses: Their roles in signaling body shape, body position and movement, and muscle force. Physiological Reviews. 2012;**92**:1651-1697

[12] Osterlund C, Liu JX, Thornell LE, Eriksson PO. Muscle spindle composition and distribution in human young masseter and biceps brachii muscles reveal early growth and maturation. Anatomical Records (Hoboken). 2011;**294**:683-693

[13] Saverino D, De Santanna A, Simone R, Cervioni S, Cattrysse E, Testa M. Observational study on the occurrence of muscle spindles in human digastric and mylohyoideus muscles. BioMed Research International. 2014;**2014**:294263

[14] Cattaneo L, Pavesi G. The facial motor system. Neuroscience and Biobehavioral Reviews. 2014;**38**: 135-159

[15] Frayne E, Coulson S, Adams R, Croxson G, Waddington G. Proprioceptive ability at the lips and jaw measured using the same psychophysical discrimination task. Experimental Brain Research. 2016;**234**:1679-1687

[16] Baumel J. Trigeminal-facial nerve communications. Archives of Otolaryngology. 1974;**99**:34-44

[17] Lazarov NE. Neurobiology of orofacial proprioception. Brain Research Reviews. 2007;**56**:362-383

[18] Monhouase S. Cranial Nerves. Functional Anatomy. Cambridge: Cambridge University Press; 2005

[19] Wilson-Pawels L, Stewart T, Akesson EJ, Spacey SD. Cranial Nerves. Third Edition. Function and Dysfunction. 3er ed. People's Medical Publishing House of China; 2010

[20] Bendella H, Spacca B, Rink S, Stoffels HJ, Nakamura M, Scaal M, et al. Anastomotic patterns of the facial parotid plexus (PP): A human cadaver study. Annals of Anatomy. 2017;**213**:52-61

[21] Monkhouse WS. The anatomy of the facial nerve. Ear, Nose, & Throat Journal. 1990;**69**:677-683, 686-7

[22] Moore KL, Dalley AF. Clinically Oriented Anatomy. 4th ed. Baltimore: Lippincott Williams & Wilkins; 1999. pp. 859-861

[23] Vacher C, Cyna-Gorse F. Motor nerves of the face. Surgical and radiologic anatomy of facial paralysis and their surgical repair. Annales de Chirurgie Plastique et Esthétique. 2015;**60**:363-369

[24] De Bonnecaze G, Vergez S, Chaput B, Vairel B, Serrano E, Chantalat E, et al. Variability in facial-muscle innervation: A comparative study based on electrostimulation and anatomical dissection. Clinical Anatomy. 2018. DOI: 10.1002/ca.23081

[25] Davis RA, Anson BJ, Budinger JM, Kurth IE. 1956 surgical anatomy of the facial nerve and parotid gland based upon a study of 350 cervicofacial halves. Surgery, Gynecology & Obstetrics. 1956;**102**:385-412

[26] Cobo JL. Neuroanatomía de la cara. Anatomía topográfica, quirúrgica, radiológica y microscópica de la inervación de la cara. Oviedo: Universidad de Oviedo; 2016

[27] Ekinci N. A study on the branching pattern of the facial nerve of children. Kaibogaku Zasshi. 1999;**74**:447-450

[28] Gataa IS, Faris BJ. Patterns and surgical significance of facial nerve branching within the parotid gland in 43 cases. Oral and Maxillofacial Surgery. 2016;**20**:161-165

[29] Shimada K, Moriyama H, Ikeda M, Tomita H, Shigihara S, Gasser RF. Peripheral communication of the facial nerve at the angle of the mouth. European Archives of Oto-Rhino-Laryngology. 1994:110-112

[30] Hwang K, Han JY, Battuvshin D, Kim DJ, Chung IH. Communication of infraorbital nerve and facial nerve: Anatomic and histologic study. The Journal of Craniofacial Surgery. 2004;**15**:88-91

[31] Hwang K, Hwang JH, Cho HJ, Kim DJ, Chung IH. Horizontal branch of the supraorbital nerve and temporal branch of the facial nerve. The Journal of Craniofacial Surgery. 2005;**16**:647-649

[32] Hwang K, Jin S, Park JH, Kim DJ, Chung IH. Relation of mental nerve with mandibular branch of the facial nerve. The Journal of Craniofacial Surgery. 2007;**18**:165-168

[33] Hwang K, Yang SC, Song JS. Communications between the trigeminal nerve and the facial nerve in the face: A systematic review. The Journal of Craniofacial Surgery. 2015;**26**:1643-1646

[34] Kwak HH, Park HD, Youn KH, Hu KS, Koh KS, Han SH, et al. Branching patterns of the facial nerve and its communication with the auriculotemporal nerve. Surgical and Radiologic Anatomy. 2004;(6):494-500

[35] Tohma A, Mine K, Tamatsu Y, Shimada K. Communication between the buccal nerve (V) and facial nerve

(VII) in the human face. Annals of Anatomy. 2004;**186**:173-178

[36] Hu KS, Kwak J, Koh KS, Abe S, Fontaine C, Kim HJ. Topographic distribution area of the infraorbital nerve. Surgical and Radiologic Anatomy. 2007;**29**:383-388

[37] Diamond M, Wartmann CT, Tubbs RS, Shoja MM, Cohen-Gadol AA, Loukas M. Peripheral facial nerve communications and their clinical implications. Clinical Anatomy. 2011;**24**:10-18

[38] Odobescu A, Williams HB, Gilardino MS. Description of a communication between the facial and zygomaticotemporal nerves. Journal of Plastic, Reconstructive & Aesthetic Surgery. 2012;**65**:1188-1192

[39] Yang HM, Won SY, Kim HJ, Hu KS. Sihler staining study of anastomosis between the facial and trigeminal nerves in the ocular area and its clinical implications. Muscle & Nerve. 2013;**48**:545-550

[40] Shoja MM, Oyesiku NM, Griessenauer CJ, Radcliff V, Loukas M, Chern JJ, et al. Anastomoses between lower cranial and upper cervical nerves: A comprehensive review with potential significance during skull base and neck operations, part I: Trigeminal, facial, and vestibulocochlear nerves. Clinical Anatomy. 2014;**27**:118-130

[41] Tansatit T, Phanchart P, Chinnawong D, Apinuntrum P, Phetudom T, Sahraoui YM. A cadaveric study of the communication patterns between the Buccal trunks of the facial nerve and the Infraorbital nerve in the Midface. The Journal of Craniofacial Surgery. 2016;**27**:214-218

[42] Cobo JL, Solé-Magdalena A, Menendez I, De Vicente JC, Vega JA. Connections between the facial and trigeminal nerves: Anatomical basis for facial muscle proprioception. JPRAS Open. 2017;**12**:9-18

[43] Namking M, Boonruangsri P, Woraputtaporn W, G€uldner FH. Communication between the facial and auriculotemporal nerves. Journal of Anatomy. 1994;**185**:421-426

[44] Yang HM, Kim HJ, Hu KS. Anatomic and histological study of great auricular nerve and its clinical implication. Journal of Plastic, Reconstructive & Aesthetic Surgery. 2015;**68**:230-236

[45] Brennan PA, Elhamshary AS, Alam P, Anand R, Ammar M. Anastomosis between the transverse cervical nerve and marginal mandibular nerve: How often does it occur? The British Journal of Oral & Maxillofacial Surgery. 2017;**55**:293-295

[46] Marur T, Tuna Y, Demirci S. Facial anatomy. Clinics in Dermatology. 2014;**32**:14-23

[47] Connor NP, Abbs JH. Orofacial proprioception: Analyses of cutaneous mechanoreceptor population properties using artificial neural networks. Journal of Communication Disorders. 1998;**31**:535-542; 553

[48] Kadanoff D. Die sensiblen Nervendigungen in der mimischen Muskulatur des Menschen. Zeitschrift für Mikroskopisch-Anatomische Forschung. 1956;**62**:1-15

[49] Stål P, Eriksson PO, Eriksson A, Thornell LE. Enzyme-histochemical differences in fibre-type between the human major and minor zygomatic and the first dorsal interosseus muscles. Archives of Oral Biology. 1987;**32**:833-841

[50] Stål P, Eriksson PO, Eriksson A. Thornell LE. Enzyme-histochemical and morphological characteristics of muscle fibre types in the human buccinator and orbicularis oris. Archives of Oral Biology. 1990;**35**:449-458

[51] Kamen G, De Luca CJ. Firing rate interactions among human orbicularis oris motor units. The International Journal of Neuroscience. 1992;**64**:167-175

[52] Happak W, Burggasser G, Liu J, Gruber H, Freilinger G. Anatomy and histology of the mimic muscles and the supplying facial nerve. European Archives of Oto-Rhino-Laryngology. 1994;**1994**:S85-S86

[53] Goodmurphy CW, Ovalle WK. Morphological study of two human facial muscles: Orbicularis oculi and corrugator supercilii. Clin Ant. 1999;**12**:1-11

[54] Cobo JL, Abbate F, de Vicente JC, Cobo J, Vega JA. Searching for proprioceptors in human facial muscles. Neuroscience Letters. 2017;**640**:1-5

[55] Nelson CC, Blaivas M. Orbicularis oculi muscle in children. Histologic and histochemical characteristics. Investigative Ophthalmology & Visual Science. 1991;**32**:646-654

[56] May A, Bramke S, Funk RHW, May CA. The human platysma contains numerous muscle spindles. Journal of Anatomy. 2018;**232**:146-151

[57] Kröger S. Propioception 2.0: Novel functions for muscle spindles. Current Opinion in Neurology. 2018;**31**:592-598

[58] Simon A, Shenton F, Hunter I, Banks RW, Bewick GS. Amiloride-sensitive channels are a major contributor to mechanotransduction in mammalian muscle spindles. The Journal of Physiology. 2010;**588**:171-185

[59] Chen CC, Wong CW. Neurosensory mechanotransduction through acid-sensing ion channels. Journal of Cellular and Molecular Medicine. 2013;**17**:337-349

[60] Gautam M, Benson CJ. Acid-sensing ion channels (ASICs) in mouse skeletal muscle afferents are heteromers composed of ASIC1a, ASIC2, and ASIC3 subunits. The FASEB Journal. 2013;**27**:793-802

[61] Woo SH, Lukacs V, de Nooij JC, Zaytseva D, Criddle CR, Francisco A, et al. Patapoutian. Piezo2 is the principal mechanotransduction channel for proprioception. Nature Neuroscience. 2015;**18**:1756-1762

Section 3

Recent Advances in the Treatment of Facial Nerve Problem

Chapter 3

Treatment of Facial Nerve Palsy Based on Genetic Analysis of the Facial Muscles

Hiroshi Moriyama

Abstract

Details of the molecular biological features of facial nerve palsy have not been widely reported in textbooks. I performed a genetic analysis of facial muscle specimens from Japanese patients with moderate (House-Brackmann facial nerve grading system III) and severe (House-Brackmann facial nerve grading system V) dysfunctions due to Bell's palsy and rats, after facial nerve resection (total paralysis). Microarray analysis of gene expression was performed using specimens from both the healthy and affected sides, and gene expressions were compared. Changes in gene expression were defined as a palsy/healthy side ratio >2.0 or <0.5. I observed changes of gene expression; in particular, genes for muscle, neuron, and energy function showed changes with the severity of facial nerve palsy. This study may aid the development of new treatments and diagnostic/prognostic markers based on the severity of palsy.

Keywords: facial nerve palsy, facial muscle, orbicularis oculi, microarray analysis, gene expression

1. Introduction

Bell's palsy is an acute, idiopathic, unilateral facial nerve paresis or paralysis of unknown cause. It leads to the partial or complete inability to voluntarily move facial muscles on the affected side of the face and may be occurring with equal frequency on the right and left sides of the face. Although typically self-limited, symptoms of Bell's palsy may include oropharyngeal or facial numbness, disturbed taste on the anterior part of the tongue, impaired tolerance to ordinary levels of noise, mild pain in or behind the ear, significant oral incompetence, and an inability to close the eyelid, leading to potential eye injury. Clinically important improvement without intervention occurs within 3 weeks after onset of symptoms in 85% of patients and within 3–5 months in the remaining 15% [1]. Patients failing to show signs of improvement by 3 weeks may have suffered Wallerian degeneration of the facial nerve, leading to residual paresis and abnormal branching of regenerating axons, or may have an alternative diagnosis that requires identification by specialist examination or investigations. Among patients with Bell's palsy, 71% obtained their normal facial muscle function [1]. Sequelae were slight in 12% of patients with Bell's palsy, mild in 13%, and severe in 4% [1]. Incomplete recovery of facial expression may have a long-term impact on quality of life. Some patients with Bell's palsy never recover despite treatment by pharmacotherapy and facial nerve decompression surgery. Physicians take the bold course of operation as a last resort. Contemporary reconstructive options include neurotization procedures (a new motor nerve is used to restore innervation to a viable muscle), contiguous regional muscle transfer (most commonly temporalis muscle transfer), and microsurgical free muscle transfer [2]. Additionally, some patients do not wish to undergo plastic and reconstructive surgery, and at present, there is no effective treatment for them [3]. Research on myogenin expression in the facial muscles following resection or compression of the facial nerve [4] indicated that facial muscle gene analysis might be a promising way to predict the outcome of facial palsy even at an early stage of the disease [4]. I thus performed a genetic analysis of the facial muscles in patients with Bell's palsy and in rats after facial nerve resection and assessed its molecular biological aspects as a pathway to new treatments.

2. Materials and methods

2.1 Human specimens

The materials used to study the microarray analysis were obtained from the orbicularis oculi muscles of six Japanese patients with Bell's palsy (females in their 60s). Three patients were judged to be House-Brackmann facial nerve grading system III (moderate dysfunction), and the other three were judged to be House-Brackmann facial nerve grading system V (severe dysfunction). Both groups had previously received nonsurgical conservative treatment using steroids and so on but had not undergone facial nerve decompression surgery. All the patients were treated with plastic and reconstructive procedures at 1.5 years after the onset of facial paralysis. Both groups underwent blepharoplasty of the superior eyelid for blepharoptosis on the affected side. They also underwent blepharoplasty on the healthy side for esthetic reasons. Biopsy materials were obtained from the palpebral part of orbicularis oculi on both the healthy side and the side with palsy. The microarray analysis of gene expression was performed using Affymetrix Human Gene 1.0 ST arrays (Affymetrix Inc., Santa Clara, CA, USA), and gene expressions were compared between the two sides. Changes of gene expression were defined as a palsy/healthy side expression ratio >2.0 or <0.5.

This study was approved by the local ethics review board (No. 149) at the Showa University Hospital. I conducted and had supervisory control of this study according to the Ethical Principles for Medical Research Involving Human Subjects in the Declaration of Helsinki. I provided all patients with detailed information about this study and obtained written informed consent prior to inclusion from both patients and doctors for participation in this study.

2.2 Rat specimens

Three male Slc: Wistar/ST rats weighing 300 g (12 weeks old) were used. The management of environmental variables of rats was as follows: (1) the room temperature range for rat housing between 21 and 23°C, (2) the humidity at the level of rat cages of 40–70%, (3) the room ventilation rates of about 15–20 air changes per hour, and (4) the light cycles of 12/12 hours light/dark. The animals were allowed to have food and water provided ad libitum until the end of the experiment.

Each animal was anesthetized with an intraperitoneal injection of 0.15 mg/kg of medetomidine hydrochloride, 2.0 mg/kg of midazolam, and 2.5 mg/kg of butorphanol tartrate and fixed on an experimental table in the prone position. The face was shaved and cleaned, and a skin incision was made to expose the extratemporal portion of the facial nerve bilaterally. On the nerve resection side (right side), the main trunk of the facial nerve was cut just distal to the stylomastoid foramen, forming a 7 mm gap in the trunk to avoid regeneration. In sham surgery group, the facial nerve on the opposite side (left side) was exposed without further manipulation. The rats were returned to the animal room after completion of these procedures.

The rats were sacrificed under deep anesthesia by intraperitoneal administration of pentobarbital (150 mg/kg) on the third postoperative week. A piece of orbicularis oculi muscle was obtained from each side and immediately immersed in RNA*later* solution (QIAGEN N. V.; Venlo, Netherlands), for gene expression analysis. The microarray analysis of gene expression was performed using Affymetrix Human Gene 1.0 ST arrays (Affymetrix Inc., Santa Clara, CA, USA), and gene expression was compared between the two sides. Changes of gene expression were defined as a palsy/healthy side expression ratio >2.0 or <0.5.

Under the approval of the Ethics Committee of Nagoya City University Graduate School of Medical Sciences (No. H27M-74), the present study was conducted following the Guidelines for Animal Experimentation at the above institute. All efforts were made to minimize suffering and the number of animals used, as described in the experimental protocol.

3. Results

Table 1 summarizes the data from the three severities of facial nerve palsy (House-Brackmann facial nerve grading system III, V, and VI). Only 13 genes showed similar changes between patients with moderate dysfunction and those with severe dysfunction, and only one gene showed similar changes between patients with moderate dysfunction and rats with total paralysis. In contrast, 333 genes showed similar changes between patients with severe dysfunction and rats with total paralysis. The overall changes indicated that patients with moderate dysfunction differed from those with severe dysfunction and rats with total paralysis.

Species	Human	Human	Rat
Severity of facial nerve palsy	Moderate dysfunction	Severe dysfunction	Total paralysis
House-Brackmann facial nerve grading system	III	V	VI
Gene category			
Muscle	↑20 ↓4	↓↓	↓↓
Neuron	↓↓	↑39 ↓20	↑29 ↓18
Energy	↑	↓↓	↓↓
Immunity	→	↑	↑
Inflammation	→	↑	↑↑
Stress	→	↑	↑
Apoptosis	→	→	→
Autophagy	→	→	↑
Death	→	→	→

Table 1.
Comparison of changes in gene expression between the three severities of facial nerve palsy. Changes of gene expression were defined as a palsy/healthy side ratio > 2.0 or < 0.5. ↓↓ *indicates that most genes in the category were downregulated.* ↓ *indicates that some genes in the category were downregulated.* ↑↑ *indicates that most genes in the category were upregulated.* ↑ *indicates that some genes in the category were upregulated.* → *indicates that expression of genes in the category did not change. Numbers (mean values) on the right side of the arrows indicate the number of genes showing changes.*

3.1 Patients with moderate dysfunction

A total of 174 genes showed changes, which was a relatively low number. Genes in the neuron category tended to show downregulation, while most genes showing changes in the muscle category were upregulated. Genes related to muscle components and genes involved in muscle movement were also upregulated. Only two energy production genes were upregulated, and both were important genes related to the glycolysis pathway. I did not find any large functional clusters except for these functional categories. Some genes involved in cell proliferation and cell division showed downregulation. However, genes linked to stress markers and apoptosis did not show upregulation (**Table 1**).

3.2 Patients with severe dysfunction

A total of 763 genes showed changes of expression. Among 59 genes with changes in the neuron category, 39 genes showed upregulation and 20 genes showed downregulation. Most genes showing changes in the muscle and energy categories showed downregulation, but some genes related to immunity, inflammation, and stress, in contrast, showed upregulation (**Table 1**).

3.3 Rats with total paralysis

A total of 1102 genes showed changes of expression. Among 47 genes with changes in the neuron category, 29 genes were upregulated and 18 were downregulated. Some genes linked to immunity, stress, and autophagy were also upregulated. Moreover, most genes showing changes in the inflammation category were upregulated. In contrast, most genes showing changes in the muscle and energy categories showed downregulation (**Table 1**).

4. Discussion

The total number of genes showing changes of expression (mean values for the patients) in the patients with moderate dysfunction was 174, compared to 763 in the patients with severe dysfunction. The total number of genes that changed in both groups was 25, but only 13 genes showed changes of expression in the same direction. Next, the total number of genes showing changes of expression (mean values for the patients and rats) in the patients with moderate dysfunction was 174 but 1102 in the rats with total paralysis. The total number of genes that changed in both groups was 19, but only one gene showed changes of expression in the same direction. These findings indicated that the condition of moderate dysfunction differed greatly from that of severe dysfunction in patients with facial nerve palsy and rats with total paralysis.

Considering these findings, I speculate that, if facial nerve conduction is reduced in moderate dysfunction, the orbicularis oculi muscle cannot function well and the patient presents with paresis. To improve this situation, regeneration of muscle tissue is promoted. Researchers reported that innervation is required for normal energy production in muscles [5]. Therefore, due to denervation, there was the decrease in energy production in muscles with paresis, but patients with moderate dysfunction had some energy production related to regeneration of muscle tissue. There was very little energy production or regeneration of the affected muscles because of the largely abolished facial nerve conduction in patients with severe dysfunction. Accordingly, the muscles innervated by the facial nerve did not show much regeneration, but the neurons themselves showed accelerated regeneration.

On the basis of these genetic findings, I suggest that neurorrhaphy and nerve grafting of the facial nerve are appropriate for patients with moderate dysfunction. These procedures will improve facial nerve conduction, leading to the increase in energy production for the regeneration of muscle tissue. However, there was little muscle regeneration and very low energy production in patients with severe dysfunction, although they showed acceleration of neuronal regeneration. These findings may explain why neurorrhaphy and nerve grafting of the facial nerve are unsuccessful if performed more than 1 year after the onset of facial palsy. Many authors have reported that recovery is better if the interval between injury to the facial nerve and repair surgery on the facial nerve is shorter [6–8]. Because improvement of facial nerve conduction is incomplete in patients with severe dysfunction, I consider that promoting the regeneration of muscle tissue and energy production is necessary. It is possible that some form of regenerative medicine, such as the use of induced pluripotent stem (iPS) cells, could be employed to improve muscle regeneration [9]. However, before such treatments become available for clinical use, I propose administration of pyruvate or mitochonic acid 5 (MA-5) as a practical way to promote muscle regeneration and energy production. Pyruvate plays a pivotal role in central carbon metabolism. Pyruvate is generated from several sources, including the end product of glycolysis, the oxidation of lactate, or as the transamination of alanine. Pyruvate is crucial for ATP generation in mitochondria and for driving several major biosynthetic pathways intersecting the citric acid cycle. In addition, it is well known that pyruvate can eliminate hydrogen peroxide by a nonenzymatic reaction to form acetate, carbon dioxide, and water [10]. This antioxidant activity of pyruvate may be also beneficial for patients with mitochondrial disorders, because the respiratory defects increase the leakage of reactive oxygen species from the mitochondria. Thus, administration of pyruvate restores the production of adenosine 5′-triposphate (ATP) via the glycolytic pathway. MA-5 targets the mitochondrial protein mitofilin at the crista junction of the inner membrane and could be a novel treatment for diseases associated with mitochondrial dysfunction [11, 12]. In Bell's palsy patients with severe dysfunction, it seems that mitochondrial cytopathy develops with impairment of ATP synthesis. As this state is similar to that in various mitochondrial diseases, I consider that pyruvate therapy [13, 14] and the administration of MA-5 could be effective. I also propose neurovascular free muscle transfer as effective surgery for patients with severe dysfunction of facial palsy. Neurovascular free muscle transfer is one of the main reconstructive surgeries for established or long-standing facial palsy [15], but it also seems to be suitable for severe facial palsy based on genetic findings in this study, and I suggest that neurovascular free muscle transfer could be more effective than facial nerve neurorrhaphy with nerve grafting in patients with severe dysfunction.

Grading of facial function is necessary for evaluating and communicating the spontaneous course and the results of medical and surgical treatment of facial palsy [16, 17]. Several grading systems for the assessment of facial nerve function using gross (e.g., the House-Brackmann grading system) [16] or regional (e.g., the Yanagihara grading system) [18] scales have been proposed. In this study, patients with severe dysfunction who were judged as grade V by the House-Brackmann system also scored 8–14 points with the Yanagihara system. The clinical description in patients with severe dysfunction is barely perceptible motion, whereas that in patients with total paralysis (House-Brackmann grading system VI) is no movement. As these two clinical descriptions differ widely, I compared the changes in gene expression between patients with severe dysfunction and rats with total paralysis (**Table 1**). The total number of genes that changed in both groups was 403 and that of gene expression in the same direction accounted for around 83% (333 genes). Some genes linked to immunity, inflammation (most genes showing changes in rats), and stress were upregulated in both groups. In the neuron category, the number of upregulated genes tended to be higher than the number of downregulated genes in both groups. Moreover, in both groups, most genes showing changes in the energy and muscle categories were downregulated. As mentioned above, the condition of moderate dysfunction differed widely from that of severe dysfunction in patients with facial nerve palsy and rats with total paralysis, but the overall changes indicated that gene expressions in patients with severe dysfunction were similar to those in rats with total paralysis. In general, the molecular biological changes after neurotmesis are as follows: (1) nerve transection produces morphological changes in the neuronal perikarya known as chromatolysis or axon reaction, and the changes include swelling of the cell body, nucleolar enlargement, displacement of the nucleus to the periphery, and dissolution of Nissl bodies [19] and (2) axotomized neurons respond by upregulation of regeneration-associated genes in association with conversion of the neuron from a transmitting to a growth state [20]. Remarkable molecular biological changes after neurotmesis, as described above, lasted for 10–20 days. Rat specimens in this study were obtained on the third postoperative week. Therefore, the rat models in this study closely resembled patients with total paralysis (House-Brackmann grading system VI). Synthesizing these results based on molecular biological analyses, I suggest that clinicians treat patients with severe dysfunction (House-Brackmann grading system V) with the same treatment as for patients with total paralysis (House-Brackmann grading system VI).

5. Conclusions

I conclude that the gene expression in facial nerve palsy changes with the degree of facial nerve palsy. This study will aid in the development of new treatments and diagnostic/prognostic markers based on the severity of facial nerve palsy.

Acknowledgements

I thank Prof. Nobuyuki Mitsukawa for providing human specimens and Prof. Shingo Murakami and Dr. Akira Inagaki for providing animal specimens. I thank Dr. Yoshiyuki Takahara for helping in analyzing the DNA microarray and Ms. Ikuko Moriyama for assistance in preparing the manuscript.

Conflicts of interest

The author has no conflicts of interest to declare.

Ethics approval of research

The local Ethics Review Board of Showa University Hospital approved the study protocol (No. 149) according to the principles of the Declaration of Helsinki. All the patients were provided with detailed information about the study and provided written informed consent prior to their inclusion. I abided by the Ethical Principles for Medical Research Involving Human Subjects outlined in the Declaration of Helsinki. With regard to animal experimentation, the present study was conducted following the Guidelines for Institutional Animal Experimentation under the approval of the Ethics Committee of Nagoya City University Graduate School of Medical Sciences (No. H27M-74). I made every effort to minimize pain, discomfort for the animals and the number of animals used, as written in the experimental protocol.

Financial support and disclosure

This work was supported by the annual budget of Showa University for scientific research. I certify that the funding agencies had no involvement in the design, data collection, analysis, or interpretation of the results. The corresponding author had full access to all the data in the study and had final responsibility for the decision to submit for publication.

Author details

Hiroshi Moriyama
Department of Anatomy, Showa University School of Medicine, Shinagawa-ku, Tokyo, Japan

*Address all correspondence to: veloce@med.showa-u.ac.jp

References

[1] Peitersen E. Bell's palsy: The spontaneous course of 2,500 peripheral facial nerve palsies of different etiologies. Acta Oto-Laryngologica. Supplementum. 2002;**549**:4-30

[2] Garcia R, Hadlock T, Klebuc M, Simpson R, Zenn M, Marcus J. Contemporary solutions for the treatment of facial nerve paralysis. Plastic and Reconstructive Surgery. 2015;**135**:1025e-1046e

[3] Holland J, Bernstein J. Bell's palsy. BMJ Clinical Evidence. 2011;**2011**:1204

[4] Teraoka M, Hato N, Takahashi H, Komobuchi H, Sawai N, Okada M, et al. Myogenin expression in facial muscle following damage to the facial nerve. Acta Oto-Laryngologica. 2012;**132**:783-787

[5] Sato D, Shinzawa G, Kusunoki M, Matsui T, Sasaki H, Feng Z, et al. Effects of electrical microstimulation of peripheral sympathetic nervous fascicle on glucose uptake in rats. Journal of Artificial Organs. 2013;**16**:352-358

[6] Conley J, Baker DC. Hypoglossal-facial nerve anastomosis for reinnervation of the paralyzed face. Plastic and Reconstructive Surgery. 1979;**63**:63-72

[7] Gavron JP, Clemis JD. Hypoglossal-facial nerve anastomosis: A review of forty cases caused by facial nerve injuries in the posterior fossa. The Laryngoscope. 1984;**94**:1447-1450

[8] Kunihiro T, Kanzaki J, Yoshihara S, Satoh Y, Satoh A. Hypoglossal-facial nerve anastomosis after acoustic neuroma resection: lnfluence of the time of anastomosis on recovery of facial movement. ORL: Journal for Otorhinolaryngology and Its Related Specialties. 1996;**58**:32-35

[9] Masumoto H, Ikuno T, Takeda M, Fukushima H, Marui A, Katayama S, et al. Human iPS cell-engineered cardiac tissue sheets with cardiomyocytes and vascular cells for cardiac regeneration. Scientific Reports. 2014;**4**:6716. DOI: 10.1038/srep06716

[10] Nath K, Ngo E, Hebbel R, Croatt A, Zhou B, Nutter L. alph-Ketoacids scavenge H2O2 in vitro and in vivo and reduce menadione-induced DNA injury and cytotoxicity. The American Journal of Physiology. 1995;**268**:C227-C236

[11] Suzuki T, Yamaguchi H, Kikusato M, Hashizume O, Nagatoishi S, Matsuo A, et al. Mitochonic acid 5 binds mitochondria and ameliorates renal tubular and cardiac myocyte damage. Journal of the American Society of Nephrology. 2016;**27**:1925-1932

[12] Suzuki T, Yamaguchi H, Kikusato M, Matsuhashi T, Matsuo A, Sato T, et al. Mitochonic acid 5 (MA-5), a derivative of the plant hormone indole-3-acetic acid, improves survival of fibroblasts from patients with mitochondrial diseases. The Tohoku Journal of Experimental Medicine. 2015;**236**:225-232

[13] Tanaka M, Nishigaki Y, Fuku N, Ibi T, Sahashi K, Koga Y. Therapeutic potential of pyruvate therapy for mitochondrial diseases. Mitochondrion. 2007;**7**:399-401

[14] Kerr DS. Review of clinical trials for mitochondrial disorders: 1997-2012. Neurotherapeutics. 2013;**10**:307-319

[15] Takushima A, Harii K, Asato H, Kurita M, Shiraishi T. Fifteen-year survey of one-stage latissimus dorsi muscle transfer for treatment of longstanding facial paralysis. Journal of Plastic, Reconstructive & Aesthetic Surgery. 2013;**66**:29-36

[16] House JW, Brackmann DE. Facial nerve grading system. Otolaryngology and Head and Neck Surgery. 1985;**93**:146-147

[17] House JW. Facial nerve grading systems. The Laryngoscope. 1983;**93**:1056-1069

[18] Yanagihara N. Grading of facial palsy. In: Fisch U, editor. Proceedings of the Third International Symposium on Facial Nerve Surgery. Zurich: Kugler Medical Publications; 1976. pp. 533-535

[19] Kreutzberg GW. Microglia, the first line of defense in brain pathologies. Arzneimittel-Forschung. 1995;**45**:357-360

[20] Boyd JG, Gordon T. Neurotrophic factors and their receptors in axonal regeneration and functional recovery after peripheral nerve injury. Molecular Neurobiology. 2003;**27**:277-324

Chapter 4

The Use of Phototherapy for Bell's Palsy

Diego Rothschild and Shu Yan Ng

Abstract

Various methods have been used to treat Bell's palsy, ranging from physical therapy, medications, to decompression surgery. The standard treatment is currently a prescription of corticosteroids with antiviral agents. All these medical approaches yield mixed results, and there is a need for additional investigation on treatment options. Recent studies have shown that facial palsy responds positively to phototherapy treatment, in particular the low-energy infrared laser. In the present report, we attempt to review the current clinical application of phototherapy, representing a conservative and safe medical approach in the treatment of Bell's palsy. A literature review was performed. The results of the included studies suggested that low-level laser therapy (LLLT) is a significant treatment modality for patients recovering from Bell's palsy. However, the risk of bias of the included studies was relatively high, and further research could change the estimate of effect of this treatment option. In conclusion, there is currently a moderate evidence to support the effectiveness of low-level laser therapy in the treatment of Bell's palsy. Further randomized double-blind placebo-controlled trials and high-quality studies are needed to determine with certainty the benefits of this treatment option for Bell's palsy.

Keywords: low-level laser therapy, infrared laser, LED, facial palsy, Bell's palsy

1. Introduction

Bell's palsy is an idiopathic lesion to the facial nerve, also known as cranial nerve VII. It is responsible for the control of the muscles of the facial mimic. It is the most common unilateral facial paralysis [1] and is diagnosed by excluding the other possible etiologies including congenital, neoplastic, tumors, diabetes mellitus, polyneuropathy, iatrogenic, infection, trauma, and other inflammatory causes [2, 3]. Bell's palsy is characterized by a rapid onset over several hours and partial or complete unilateral paralysis of the facial nerve without other neurologic complaints [4, 5].

This paralysis is related to an inflammation of the facial nerve near the stylomastoid foramen. The main sign for Bell's palsy is a distorted facial expression, but patients can experience other symptoms (e.g., taste loss, pain around the ear, or hearing problems [2, 6]).

With an incidence oscillating between 11 and 40 cases per 100,000 inhabitants per year [7–9], Bell's palsy represents a relatively common disease that raises important psychological issues because it involves the ability to express emotions, and a diminished facial expression interferes with social interactions [10]. Indeed, the face represents psychologically the most important part of the body and an important component of self-concept [11].

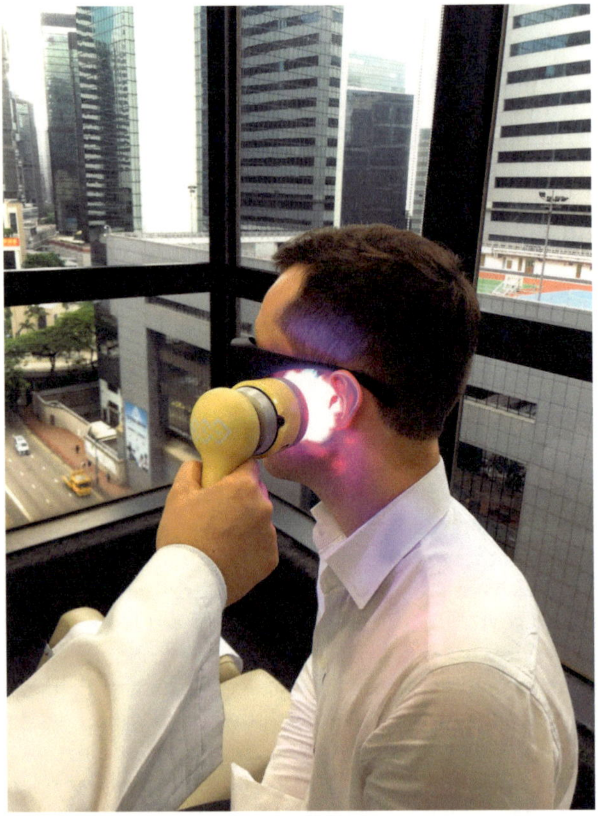

Figure 1.
Patient receiving low-level laser therapy treatment for Bell's palsy.

Concerning the prognosis, some studies show that complete recovery from Bell's palsy occurs in 70–85% of affected patients, whereas the remaining 15–30% demonstrate incomplete recovery with symptoms such as weakness, hyperkinesia, and synkinetic contracture [12–14]. As for its treatment, the standard approach is currently a prescription of corticosteroids with antiviral agents, but there are other treatment options available such as surgery and physical therapy. The use of corticosteroids has shown opposing results in different studies. Some clinical trials showed a significant benefit from treating Bell's palsy with corticosteroids [14–17]. Devriese et al. [18], however, demonstrated that its use has no significant effect on the outcome of this condition. As reported by the most reliable studies, antivirals have not been proved to be superior to placebo [19], surgery is disputed [17], and there are only a few controlled clinical trials for the efficacy of physical therapy, massage, and facial exercises.

In this context, there is a need for additional investigation on other treatment options. Recent studies have shown that facial palsy responds positively to phototherapy treatment, in particular the low-energy infrared laser. In the present report, we attempt to review the current clinical application of phototherapy, representing a conservative and safe medical approach in the treatment of Bell's palsy (**Figure 1**).

2. Low-level laser therapy and its biological effects

Lasers (light amplification by stimulated emission of radiation) were originally described in the 1960s by Theodore Maiman [20]. Seven years later Mester et al. started to investigate on low-level laser [21] and its therapeutic effects.

Low-level laser therapy involves exposing cells or tissue to low levels of red and near-infrared light, to promote tissue regeneration, reduce inflammation, and relieve pain. It is referred to as "low level" because the energy densities are low when compared to other forms of laser therapy that are used for ablation, cutting, and thermally coagulating tissue [22]. LLLT is also known as "cold laser" therapy as the power densities used are lower than those needed to produce heating of tissue.

LLLT has a photochemical effect which means the light is absorbed and causes a biochemical change [23], but the precise mechanism is not well established. From observation, it appears that LLLT has several effects at the tissue, cellular, and even molecular levels. Furthermore, different applications may change its specific modes of action. At the cellular level, existing evidence suggests that LLLT acts on the mitochondria [24], stimulates the production of adenosine triphosphate (ATP) [25], modulates the reactive oxygen species (ROS), and which then activates the transcription factors [26].

These transcription factors, in turn, induce protein synthesis that generates further effects subsequently. These effects include increase of cell propagation and migration, modulation in cytokines levels, inflammatory mediators and growth factors, and augmented tissue oxygenation [27].

The mechanisms described above only partly explain the overall effects of LLLT. This therapy has also shown to cause vasodilation, probably related to photodissociation of nitric oxide (NO) [28], which is a powerful vasodilator. This leads to better oxygenation of the targeted cells and also allows increased traffic of immune cells into tissues. Both mechanisms are linked to a faster healing.

3. Anatomy, mechanism, and etiology of Bell's palsy

In order to understand the pathophysiology of Bell's palsy and deduce the hypothetical benefits of LLLT on this condition, it is essential to know the course and function of the facial nerve (CN VII).

3.1 Anatomy

CN VII is responsible for the motor innervation of the facial muscles, stapedius, and posterior belly of the digastric muscles [29]. The facial nerve enters the temporal bone at the internal acoustic meatus and then continues along the fallopian canal before exiting through the stylomastoid foramen. It is to note that the thinnest portion of the fallopian canal is located in the internal auditory canal, at its lateral end [29].

3.2 Mechanism

The mechanism of Bell's palsy is thought to be an inflammation of CN VII with a related compression in the narrow portion of the fallopian canal [30, 31]. This inflammation causes temporary loss of motor and sensory function and potentially also leads to nerve degeneration in the longer term [30].

3.3 Etiology

The cause of this neuropathy has not been firmly established, and several theories have been proposed. One describes Bell's palsy as a mononeuritic variant of Guillain-Barre syndrome [32–34], both pathologies representing an inflammatory demyelinating neuritis.

Recent studies have linked Bell's palsy to the reactivation of latent herpes virus in the geniculate ganglia, with migration to CN VII [35, 36]. Herpes zoster virus

(HZV) and herpes simplex virus 1 (HSV-1) could be related agents, with HZV thought to be more harmful as it disseminates over the nerve via satellite cells [35]. Concerning HSV-1, its DNA has even been extracted from the endoneural fluid of CN VII during a study from a patient suffering from acute Bell's palsy [37]. Other recent studies have also shown evidence for the theory of inflammation caused by herpes simplex virus, related to nerve compression and paralysis of the face [14, 36, 38].

A correlation was also found between Bell's palsy and the inactivated intranasal influenza vaccine, with a risk multiplied by 19 for patients having received the flu vaccine as compared to that of control groups without vaccination [39]. It is of note that the peak incidence of the condition was at 31–60 days after vaccination, suggesting that an autoimmune disorder or reactivation of HSV rather than a direct toxic effect from the vaccine is operative [40]. This vaccine is no longer in use.

Other infectious etiologies that have been documented include Epstein-Barr virus, rubella, mumps, influenza, Coxsackievirus, adenovirus, cytomegalovirus, and rickettsia, with the latter being a rare cause [41, 42].

There are also noninfectious causes that have been suggested, including familial origin, with some 4–8% of patients reporting to have family history of the pathology [43], ischemia associated to atherosclerosis causing edema of the facial nerve [44–46], and autoimmune processes such as Hashimoto's encephalopathy [47, 48].

4. Effectiveness of LLLT for Bell's palsy

A literature review was performed to assess the effectiveness of LLLT for the treatment of Bell's palsy.

4.1 Method

4.1.1 Search strategy

An initial electronic search was constructed to identify English language studies that examined LLLT for Bell's palsy. PubMed, EMBASE, PEDro, and J-Stage databases were searched from inception to July 2018. The titles and abstracts have been screened in order to identify the relevant studies. Full-text copies of these studies were retrieved and considered for inclusion in this review.

4.1.2 Selection criteria

Studies were included if they were randomized and nonrandomized controlled trials evaluating the effectiveness of LLLT compared to other common interventions or compared to a placebo/sham control in the treatment of Bell's palsy. Studies were excluded if they are published in languages other than English.

4.1.3 Assessment of risk of bias for included studies

The risk of bias was assessed using the Cochrane Bias Methods Group's criteria for randomized controlled trials [49] and the Effective Practice and Organization of Care's criteria for nonrandomized trials [50].

4.1.4 Data analysis

The data was extracted and reported qualitatively only, due to the heterogeneity of the studies.

4.1.5 Grading the strength of evidence

Strength of evidence was assessed using the GRADE Working Group grades of evidence [51] as follows:

- High quality: further research is very unlikely to change our confidence in the estimate of effect.
- Moderate quality: further research is likely to have an important impact on our confidence in the estimate of effect and may change the estimate.
- Low quality: further research is very likely to have an important impact on our confidence in the estimate of effect and is likely to change the estimate.

4.2 Results

4.2.1 Study selection

The electronic search and screening of titles and abstracts identified nine potentially relevant studies; they were retrieved and considered for inclusion [52–60]. Of these studies, five satisfied the eligibility criteria and were included in the review [52–56].

4.2.2 Study characteristics

Table 1 displays the included studies' characteristics. Three studies were randomized controlled trials, and the other two were nonrandomized controlled trials. All studies compared LLLT to other common treatments (group control). Only one study [52] included a sham/placebo laser associated to a common treatment, and LLLT associated to the same treatment was compared. Two studies compared the effectiveness of LLLT and facial exercise [52, 54]. Two studies compared LLLT with corticosteroids [53, 56]. One assessed the effectiveness of LLLT in comparison to stellate ganglion block (local anesthetic injection in the sympathetic nerve tissue of the neck). Treatments varied substantially in their dosage and length, from 30 days [55] to 8.9 weeks [56]. The study samples comprised of 51, 50, 46, 52, and 24 subjects. Finally, the outcome measurement procedures consisted in different recognized scales for the assessment of facial palsy severity. One study, however [53] also included electroneurography as one of the outcome measures.

4.2.3 Risk of bias assessment

Table 2 displays the risk of bias assessment across the included studies. One randomized controlled trial (RCT) [52] was found to be overall at low risk of bias. With that exception, all other studies were at high risk of performance bias, as no sham/placebo laser procedure was established, and therefore there was no blinding of participants. The two nonrandomized controlled trials [55, 56] had high risk of selection bias as opposed to the randomized controlled trials that appeared to be

Study	Design	Study sample	Intervention	Outcome measures	Follow-up period	Outcome
Alayat et al. [52]	Randomized controlled trial	51 subjects with unilateral Bell's palsy mean age = 43 ± 9.8 years	1. HILT + facial massage and exercise 2. LLLT + facial massage and exercise 3. Facial massage and exercise	Facial disability scale, House-Brackmann scale	6 weeks	HILT and LLLT + facial massage and exercises, respectively, more effective than facial massage and exercises with sham laser
Kudoh et al. [53]	Randomized controlled trial	50 subjects with Bell's palsy age ranged from 35 to 60 years	1. LLLT + corticosteroids 2. Corticosteroids	Yanagihara evaluation scale, electroneurography (ENoG)	3 months	LLLT + corticosteroids more effective than corticosteroids alone
Ordahan et al. [54]	Randomized controlled trial	46 subjects with unilateral Bell's palsy mean age 41 ± 9.7 years	1. LLLT + facial exercise 2. Facial exercise	Facial disability index	6 weeks	LLLT + facial exercise more effective than facial exercise alone
Murakami et al. [55]	Nonrandomized controlled trial	52 subjects with Bell's palsy age ranged from 37.1 to 49.4 years	1. Stellate ganglion block (SGB) 2. LLLT 3. LLLT + SGB	Scale for assessment of facial palsy	>30 days	LLLT + SGB as effective as SGB or LLLT alone, LLLT alone shows however faster improvement
Yamada et al. [56]	Nonrandomized controlled trial	24 subjects with Hunt's syndrome II or Bell's palsy age ranged from 31.1 to 59.1	1. LLLT 2. LLLT + corticosteroids 3. Corticosteroids	Scale for assessment of facial palsy	5.3–8.9 weeks	LLLT as effective as corticosteroids, combination most effective

Table 1.
Characteristics of included studies

Study	Random sequence generation (selection bias)	Allocation concealment (selection bias)	Blinding of participants (performance bias)	Blinding of outcome assessment (detection bias)	Incomplete outcome data (attrition bias)	Other sources of bias
Alayat et al. [52]	–	–	–	–	–	–
Kudoh et al. [53]	–	?	+	+	–	–
Ordahan et al. [54]	–	–	+	+	–	–
Murakami et al. [55]	+	+	+	+	–	–
Yamada et al. [56]	+	+	+	–	–	+
+, high risk of bias; –, low risk of bias;?, undetermined.						

Table 2.
Risk of bias across the included studies

at low risk, with one study however [53] having unclear concealment in allocation. Concerning the detection bias, only two studies had a defined strategy for blinding of outcome assessment [52, 56], and the other ones therefore appeared to be at high risk of bias [53–55]. Finally, all studies were found to be at low risk of attrition bias. No other sources of bias were found, except the low number of participants in one of the studies [56].

4.2.4 LLLT effectiveness

Two studies [52, 54] showed that LLLT combined with facial exercise is more effective than facial exercise alone or in combination with a placebo laser. One study [53] found that LLLT combined with corticosteroids was more effective than corticosteroids alone, and another one [56] found that they are equally effective when prescribed separately but better when combined. Finally, the last study's [55] results support that LLLT is as effective as stellate ganglion block or the combination, but LLLT alone shows faster effects.

4.2.5 Adverse events

Three of the included studies [53, 55, 56] specify that no side effects were noted following the LLLT.

4.2.6 Overall strength of the evidence

The overall strength of the evidence was moderate. Most studies did not include patient blinding [53–56]. Moreover, three of the five studies [53–55] did not proceed to a blinding of outcome assessment which substantially increases the risk of bias. Overall, only one study [52] showed low risk of bias and high-quality evidence. In other words, further research is likely to have an important impact and may change our confidence in the estimate of effect of LLLT for the treatment of Bell's palsy.

4.3 Discussion

This literature review was conducted to investigate the effectiveness of LLLT for the treatment of Bell's palsy. In the included studies, usual treatments such as facial exercise and corticosteroids were found to be less effective alone than when combined to LLLT [52–54, 56]. Moreover, isolated LLLT and corticosteroid treatments were compared and found to be equally effective [56]. This suggests that LLLT is a significant treatment modality for patients recovering from Bell's palsy. However, the lack of outcome assessment blinding [53–55] and patient blinding [53–56] in most studies meant that the risk of bias was relatively high and further research could change the estimate of effect of this treatment option. Only one study [52] showed low risk of bias and high-quality evidence (randomized double-blind placebo-controlled trial).

The understanding of the pathophysiology of Bell's palsy helps deduce the related hypothetical benefits of LLLT. The physiological changes related to this condition have been identified during a histopathological study of the facial nerve over the acute pathological phase and included infiltration of inflammatory cells, marked edema and myelin breakdown, as well as axonal changes [61].

The photochemical and physiological changes produced by LLLT when applied onto the involved site in patients affected by Bell's palsy include increase of cell propagation and migration, modulation in cytokines levels, inflammatory mediators and growth factors, and augmented tissue oxygenation [27]. They also include vasodilation related to photodissociation of nitric oxide (NO) [28], thus leading to further oxygenation of the targeted cells and allowing increased traffic of immune cells into tissues.

In line with these changes, we can assume that LLLT helps in controlling and reducing the inflammation, swelling, and edema causing compression of the facial nerve in its bony canal. It probably also helps improve the affected nerve's function. We can also hypothesize that the augmented influx of immune cells helps fight the potential causative infectious agent.

Several studies support each one of these theories individually. Whether in fighting infectious agents such as herpes simplex virus [62], reducing inflammatory infiltrate [63], reducing edema [64], or helping nerve function and recovery [65], LLLT has shown promising results.

Furthermore, with some studies showing that complete healing occurs in 70–85% of affected patients and the remaining 15–30% demonstrates incomplete recovery (weakness, hyperkinesia, and synkinetic contracture) [12–14], Bell's palsy becomes an often unpredictable pathology, and spontaneous recovery cannot be expected. Further literature refers to a 25% of affected people with incomplete recovery with traditional medicines and therapies and retaining remarkable sequel of the pathology that may have been avertible with complementary laser treatment within 15 days of diagnosis [66].

In conclusion, LLLT seems to be a good complementary medium reducing the possibility of side effects related to facial paralysis and allowing nerve recovery. In addition, it is painless, has no adverse effects, and is suitable for all type of patients, especially those who cannot use corticosteroids, such as diabetics and hypertensive patients [66].

5. Conclusion

There is currently a moderate evidence to support the effectiveness of low-level laser therapy in the treatment of Bell's palsy. The results of the included studies suggest that LLLT may be a promising and safe treatment for this condition, but most of these studies were at substantial risk of bias. Further well-designed randomized double-blind placebo-controlled trials and high-quality studies are needed to determine with certainty the benefits of this treatment option for Bell's palsy.

Conflict of interest

The authors declare that they have no conflict of interest.

Abbreviation

LLLT	low-level laser therapy
ATP	adenosine triphosphate
ROS	reactive oxygen species
NO	nitric oxide
CN VII	facial nerve
HZV	herpes zoster virus
HSV-1	herpes simplex virus 1
SGB	stellate ganglion block

Author details

Diego Rothschild* and Shu Yan Ng
Hong Kong Chiropractic College Foundation, Wanchai, Hong Kong

*Address all correspondence to: rothschild.dc@gmail.com

References

[1] Cha CI, Hong CK, Park MS, Yeo SG. Comparison of facial nerve paralysis in adults and children. Yonsei Medical Journal. 2008;**49**(5):725-734

[2] Facer GW. Facial nerve paralysis: Is it always Bell's palsy? Postgraduate Medicine. 1981;**69**:206-208, 211-213, 216

[3] Musani MA, Farooqui AN, Usman A, et al. Association of herpes simplex virus infection and Bell's palsy. JPMA. Journal of the Pakistan Medical Association. 2009;**59**(12):823-825

[4] Danner CJ. Facial nerve paralysis. Otolaryngologic Clinics of North America. 2008;**41**:619-632

[5] Tiemstra JD, Khatkhate N, Tiemstra JD, Khatkhate N. Bell's palsy: Diagnosis and management. American Family Physician. 2007;**76**(7):997-1002

[6] Sajadi MM, Sajadi MR, Tabatabaie SM. The history of facial palsy and spasm: Hippocrates to Razi. Neurology. 2011;**77**:174-178

[7] De Diego-Sastre JI, Prim-Espada MP, Fernández-García F. The epidemiology of Bell's palsy. Revista de Neurologia. 2005;**41**(5):287-290

[8] Morris AM, Deeks SL, Hill MD, Midroni G, Goldstein WC, Mazzulli T, et al. Annualized incidence and spectrum of illness from an outbreak investigation of Bell's palsy. Neuroepidemiology. 2002;**21**(5):255-261

[9] Tovi F, Hadar T, Sidi J, Sarov I, Sarov B. Epidemiological aspects of idiopathic peripheral facial palsy. European Journal of Epidemiology. 1986;**2**(3):228-232

[10] Bradbury ET, Simons W, Sanders R. Psychological and social factors in reconstructive surgery for hemi-facial palsy. Journal of Plastic, Reconstructive & Aesthetic Surgery. 2006;**59**:272-278

[11] Ho AL, Scott AM, Klassen AF, Cano SJ, Pusic AL, Van Laeken N. Measuring quality of life and patient satisfaction in facial paralysis patients: A systematic review of patient-reported outcome measures. Plastic and Reconstructive Surgery. 2012;**130**(1):91-99

[12] Yanagihara N. Incidence of Bell's palsy. Annals of Otology, Rhinology and Laryngology. 1988;**97**(Suppl 137):3-4

[13] Koike Y, Imamura H. Effects of early administration high-dose steroids on Bell's palsy. In: Castro D, editor. The Facial Nerve. Amstelveen: Kuger and Ghedini Publ; 1990. pp. 395-400

[14] Peitersen E. Bell's palsy: The spontaneous course of 2,500 peripheral facial nerve palsies of different etiologies. Acta Oto-Laryngologica. Supplementum. 2002;**549**:4-30

[15] Ilniczky S, Semmelweis E, Altalános Orvostudományi K, Neurológiai K. Clinical analysis of patients with peripheral facial palsy. Ideggyógyászati Szemle. 2006;**59**(11-12):400-405

[16] Glass GE, Tzafetta K. Bell's palsy: A summary of current evidence and referral algorithm. Family Practice. 2014. pii: cmu058

[17] Hohman MH, Hadlock TA. Etiology, diagnosis, and management of facial palsy: 2000 patients at a facial nerve center. The Laryngoscope. 2014;**124**(7):E283-E293. DOI: 10.1002/lary.24542

[18] Devriese PP, Schumacher T, Scheide A, DeJongh RH, Houtkooper JM. Incidence, prognosis and recovery of Bell's palsy. A survey about 1000 patients (1974-1983). Clinical Otolaryngology. 1990;**15**:15-27

[19] Sullivan FM, Swan IR, Donnan PT, Morrison JM, Smith BH, et al. Early treatment with prednisolone

or acyclovir in Bell's palsy. The New England Journal of Medicine. 2007;**357**(16):1598-1607

[20] Maiman TH. Stimulated optical radiation in ruby. Nature. 1960;**187**:493-494

[21] Mester E, Szende B, Tora JG. Effect of laser on hair growth of mice. Kísérletes Orvostudomány. 1967;**19**:628-631

[22] Hamblin MR. Mechanisms of low level light therapy. Proceedings of SPIE. 2009;**6140**:614001-614001

[23] Huang YY, Chen AC, Carroll JD, Hamblin MR. Biphasic dose response in low level light therapy. Dose-Response. 2009;**7**(4):358-383

[24] Greco M, Guida G, Perlino E, Marra E, Quagliariello E. Increase in RNA and protein synthesis by mitochondria irradiated with helium-neon lase. Biochemical and Biophysical Research Communications. 1989;**163**:1428-1434

[25] Karu TI. Primary and secondary mechanisms of action of visible to near-IR radiation on cells. Journal of Photochemistry and Photobiology. B. 1999;**49**:1-17

[26] Chen AC-H, Arany PR, Huang Y-Y, Tomkinson EM, Saleem T, Yull FE, et al. Low level laser therapy activates NF-κB via generation of reactive oxygen species in mouse embryonic fibroblasts. Proceedings of SPIE. 2009;**7165**:71650-71659

[27] Karu TI, Kolyakov SF. Exact action spectra for cellular responses relevant to phototherapy. Photomedicine and Laser Surgery. 2005;**23**:355-361

[28] Lohr NL, Keszler A, Pratt P, Bienengraber M, Warltier DC, Hogg N. Enhancement of nitric oxide release from nitrosyl hemoglobin and nitrosyl myoglobin by red/near infrared radiation: Potential role in cardioprotection. Journal of Molecular and Cellular Cardiology. 2009;**47**:256-263

[29] Runge MS, Greganti MA. Netter's Internal Medicine. 2nd ed. Philadelphia (PA): Elsevier; 2009

[30] Jackson CG, von Doersten PG. The facial nerve. Current trends in diagnosis, treatment, and rehabilitation. The Medical Clinics of North America. 1999;**83**(1):179-195

[31] Liu J, Li Y, Yuan X, Lin Z. Bell's palsy may have relations to bacterial infection. Medical Hypotheses. 2009;**72**(2):169-170

[32] Aviel A, Ostfeld E, Burstein R, Marshak G, Bentwich Z. Peripheral blood T and B lymphocyte subpopulations in Bell's palsy. The Annals of Otology, Rhinology, and Laryngology. 1983;**92**(2 Pt 1):187-191

[33] Greco A, Gallo A, Fusconi M, Marinelli C, Macri GF, de Vincentiis M. Bell's palsy and autoimmunity. Autoimmunity Reviews. 2012;**12**(2):323-328

[34] Chaco J. Subclinical peripheral nerve involvement in unilateral Bell's palsy. American Journal of Physical Medicine. 1973;**52**(4):195-197

[35] Holland NJ, Weiner GM. Recent developments in Bell's palsy. BMJ. 2004;**329**(7465):553-557

[36] Schirm J, Mulkens PS. Bell's palsy and herpes simplex virus. APMIS. 1997;**105**(11):815-823

[37] Murakami S, Mizobuchi M, Nakashiro Y, Doi T, Hato N, Yanagihara N. Bell palsy and herpes simplex virus: Identification of viral DNA in endoneurial fluid and muscle. Annals of Internal Medicine. 1996;**124**(1 Pt 1):27-30

[38] Baringer JR. Herpes simplex virus and Bell palsy. Annals of Internal Medicine. 1996;**124**(1 Pt 1):63-65

[39] Mutsch M, Zhou W, Rhodes P, Bopp M, Chen RT, Linder T, et al. Use of the inactivated intranasal influenza vaccine and the risk of Bell's palsy in Switzerland. The New England Journal of Medicine. 2004;**350**(9):896-903

[40] Couch RB. Nasal vaccination, escherichia coli enterotoxin, and Bell's palsy. The New England Journal of Medicine. 2004;**350**(9):860-861

[41] Morgan M, Nathwani D. Facial palsy and infection: The unfolding story. Clinical Infectious Diseases. 1992;**14**(1):263-271

[42] Bitsori M, Galanakis E, Papadakis CE, Sbyrakis S. Facial nerve palsy associated with Rickettsia conorii infection. Archives of Disease in Childhood. 2001;**85**(1):54-55

[43] Wolfson AB. Narwood-Nuss' Clinical Practice of Emergency Medicine. 5th ed. Philadelphia (PA): Lippincott Williams & Williams; 2009

[44] Goroll AH, Mulley AG. Primary Care Medicine: Office Evaluation and Management of the Adult Patient. 6th ed. Lippincott Williams & Williams: Philadelphia (PA); 2009

[45] Merwarth HR. The occurence of peripheral facial paralysis in hypertension vascular disease. Annals of Internal Medicine. 1942;**17**:298-230

[46] Raff MC, Asbury AK. Ischemic mononeuropathy and mononeuropathy multiplex in diabetes mellitus. The New England Journal of Medicine. 1968;**279**(1):17-21

[47] Schaitkin BM, May M, Podvinec M, et al. Idiopathic (Bell's) palsy, herpes zoster cephalicus, and other facial nerve disorders of viral origin. In: May M, Schaitkin BM, editors. The Facial Nerve: May's. 2nd ed. New York: Thieme Medical; 2000. pp. 319-338

[48] He L, Li M, Long XH, Li XP, Peng Y. A case of Hashimoto's encephalopathy misdiagnosed as viral encephalitis. American Journal of Case Reports. 2013;**14**:366-369

[49] JPT H, Green S. Cochrane Handbook for Systematic Reviews of Interventions. Chichester, England: John Wiley & Sons Ltd; 2011. (Version 5.1.0): Chapter 8

[50] Cochrane Effective Practice and Organisation of Care. EPOC–specific resources for review authors. 2016. Available at: http://epoc.cochrane.org/resources/epoc-resources-review-authors. [Accessed: June 10, 2016]

Andrews JC, Schünemann HJ, Oxman AD, et al. GRADE guidelines: 15. Going from evidence to recommendation–determinants of a recommendation's direction and strength. Journal of Clinical Epidemiology. 2013;**66**(7):726-735

[51] Mohamed A, Ahmed ES, Amir E-F. Efficacy of high and low level laser therapy in the treatment of Bell's palsy: A randomized double blind placebo-controlled trial. Lasers in Medical Science. 2014;**29**(1):335-342. DOI: 10.1007/ s10103-013-1352- z

[52] Kudoh A, Yodono M, Ishihara H, Matsuki A. Linear polarized light therapy improves Bell's palsy. Laser Therapy. 1998;**10**(2):65-69. Released july 05, 2011, Online ISSN 1884-7269, Print ISSN 0898-5901

[53] Banu O, Ali K. Role of low level laser therapy added to facial expression exercises in patients with idiopathic facial (Bell's) palsy. Lasers in Medical Science. 2017;**32**(4):931-936. DOI: 10.1007/ s10103-017-2195-9

[54] Murakami F, Kemmotsu O, Kawano Y, Matsumura C, Kaseno S, Imai M. Diode low reactive level laser therapy and stellate ganglion block compared In the treatment of facial palsy. Laser Therapy. 1993;**5**(3):131-135. Released April 18, 2012, Online ISSN 1884-7269, Print ISSN 0898-5901

[55] Yamada H, Yamanaka Y, Orihara H, Ogawa H. A preliminary clinical study comparing the effect of low level laser therapy (Lllt) and corticosteroid therapy In the treatment of facial palsy. Laser Therapy. 1995;**7**(4):157-162. Released January 11, 2012, Online ISSN 1884-7269, Print ISSN 0898-5901

[56] Ng SY, Chu MHE. Treatment of Bell's palsy using monochromatic infrared energy: A report of 2 cases. Journal of Chiropractic Medicine. 2014;**13**(2):96-103. DOI: 10.1016/j.jcm.2014.06.010

[57] Okuni I, Harada T, Ushigome N, Ohshiro T, Musya Y, Maruyama Y, et al. Low level laser therapy (LLLT) for facial palsy patients. Laser Therapy. 2008;**17**:135-139. DOI: 10.5978/islsm.17.135

[58] Rubis LM. Chiropractic management of Bell palsy with low level laser and manipulation: A case report. Journal of Chiropractic Medicine. 2013;**12**(4):288-291. DOI: 10.1016/j.jcm.2013.10.001

[59] Yoshida K. Lllt for facial palsy. Laser Therapy. 2010;**19**:167-169. DOI: 10.5978/islsm.19.167

[60] Linder T, Bossart W, Bodmer D. Bell's palsy and herpes simplex virus: Fact or mystery. Otology & Neurotology. 2005;**26**:109

[61] Schindl A, Neumann R. Low-intensity laser therapy is an effective treatment for recurrent herpes simplex infection. Results from a randomized double-blind placebo-controlled study. The Journal of Investigative Dermatology. 1999;**113**(2):221-223

[62] Paiva-Oliveira EL, Lima NC, Silva PH, et al. Low-level laser therapy (LLLT) reduces inflammatory infiltrate and enhances skeletal muscle repair: Histomorphometric parameters. Laser Physics. 2012;**22**:1425

[63] Stergioulas A. Low-level laser treatment can reduce edema in second degree ankle sprains. Journal of Clinical Laser Medicine & Surgery. 2004;**22**(2):125-128

[64] Rochkind S, Drory V, Alon M, Nissan M, Ouaknine GE. Laser phototherapy (780 nm), a new modality in treatment of long-term incomplete peripheral nerve injury: A randomized double-blind placebo-controlled study. Photomedicine and Laser Surgery. 2007;**25**:436-442. DOI: 10.1089/pho.2007.2093

[65] Bernal G. Helium neon and diode laser therapy is an effective adjunctive therapy for facial paralysis. Laser Therapy. 1993;**5**:79-87